THE GLP-1 TROUBLESHOOTING GUIDE

Science-Based Solutions for Semaglutide, Tirzepatide, and Other GLP-1s for Slow Responders, Plateaus, and When Results Stall

by David Brant

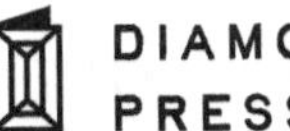

DIAMOND DOOR PRESS

Medical Disclaimer

This book is for informational and educational purposes only and does NOT provide medical advice. The author is not a physician, medical professional, or licensed healthcare provider. Nothing in this book should be construed as medical advice, diagnosis, or treatment recommendations.

GLP-1 medications are prescription drugs that require medical supervision. You must work with a qualified healthcare provider for all decisions related to your medication, including dosing, side effects, and treatment changes. Do not adjust your medication or treatment plan based on information in this book without consulting your doctor.

Always seek the advice of your physician or other qualified healthcare provider before making any changes to your diet, exercise routine, supplement regimen, or medication schedule. Never disregard professional medical advice or delay seeking it because of something you have read in this book.

The strategies and information presented are based on general fitness principles, research, and observation. They are not personalized medical recommendations. Individual results will vary significantly based on numerous factors including genetics, health status, and adherence.

If you experience concerning symptoms, side effects, or medical issues while taking GLP-1 medications, contact your healthcare provider immediately.

The author and publisher expressly disclaim any liability, loss, or risk, personal or otherwise, incurred as a consequence, directly or indirectly, of the use and application of any content in this book.

Published by Diamond Door Press
New York, NY

Printed in the United States of America

First Edition

ISBN: 978-1-971159-15-7

diamonddoorpress.com

Contents=

Introduction

You picked up this book for a reason.

Maybe you started taking a GLP-1 medication a few months ago with high hopes, and the results just haven't been what you expected. Maybe you lost some weight at first, but now the scale hasn't budged in weeks. Or maybe you're watching friends or people online talk about their amazing results, and you're wondering why your experience has been so different.

If any of that sounds familiar, you're in the right place.

The truth is, GLP-1 medications like Ozempic, Wegovy, Zepbound, and Mounjaro have helped millions of people lose weight and improve their health. They're powerful tools. But they don't work the same way for everyone. Some people see dramatic results right away. Others have a slower response. And some hit frustrating plateaus even though they're doing everything their doctor told them to do.

If you're in that second or third group, it's easy to feel like you're doing something wrong. Like maybe you're the problem. But here's what I've learned from working with hundreds of clients on these medications. You're not the problem. There are just some pieces of the puzzle that haven't clicked into place yet. And that's what this book is here to help you figure out.

Why I Wrote This Book

I've been a personal trainer for over two decades, and in the last few years, I've watched something pretty incredible happen. Clients who had been struggling with weight loss for years, sometimes decades, suddenly had access to medications that actually worked. GLP-1 medications like Ozempic, Wegovy, and Mounjaro have genuinely changed a lot of lives.

And it wasn't just my clients. I saw it happen with friends and family too. My cousin lost sixty pounds on semaglutide and finally got her blood sugar under control. A close friend who had tried what felt like every diet out there dropped three pant sizes and told me she felt like herself again for the first time in years. Watching people I care about get their health back has been really amazing.

But I also started noticing something else. Not everyone was having the same experience.

Some people would start their medication and the weight would just come off. They felt great, they had energy, everything seemed to click. But others would lose a little bit at first and then nothing. Some would do well for a few months and then hit a wall. And there were people who barely saw any results at all, even though they were following their doctor's instructions exactly.

The confusing part was that they were all on the same medications. Sometimes even the same doses. But the outcomes were completely different.

I kept hearing the same questions. Why isn't this working for me? What am I doing wrong? Is there something else I should be trying? And honestly, a lot of people felt embarrassed to even ask. They felt like they were somehow failing at something that was supposed to be easy. Like if everyone else could lose weight on these medications, what was wrong with them?

That feeling really stuck with me. Because I knew from working with these people that nothing was wrong with them. They weren't lazy. They weren't doing anything wrong. But there were often small things that were getting in the way of their results. Things that nobody had explained to them.

So I started digging deeper. I read everything I could find about how these medications work. I talked to doctors and nutritionists and other trainers. And most importantly, I worked really closely with my clients who were on GLP-1s, trying to figure out what made the difference between someone who had great results and someone who didn't.

What I learned is that these medications are powerful, but they're not magic. They do an amazing job of suppressing your appetite. That's a huge deal. But appetite suppression by itself doesn't automatically mean weight loss. Your body is complex, and weight loss depends on multiple factors working together. Things like genetics, thyroid function, and conditions like PCOS can all affect how you respond. Nutrition matters, particularly getting enough protein to protect your muscle. Movement matters. Sleep and stress matter. And yes, overall energy balance matters too. When any of these pieces are out of alignment, progress can stall. The good news is that most of these factors are things you can work with and adjust. That's what makes the difference between feeling stuck and actually seeing results.

The thing is, most people don't realize that. They think the medication will handle everything. And when it doesn't, they blame themselves.

Now, I want to be really clear about something right up front. I'm a personal trainer. I'm not a doctor. I can't give you medical advice, and I'm not going to try. This book isn't about telling you what to do with your medication. How much to take, when to take it, whether to switch to something else. Those are decisions for you and your doctor to make together.

What I can help you with is everything else. The nutrition side. The exercise side. The daily habits that can either support your medication or work against it. That's my area. And honestly, that's where a lot of people get stuck.

Think of it this way. Your doctor is managing the medication part. This book is your guide for optimizing everything around it. Both pieces matter if you want to see the best results possible.

I wrote this book because I kept having the same conversations over and over. A client or a friend would come to me frustrated and confused, wondering why the medication wasn't working for them like it seemed to work for everyone else. And almost every time, we'd find something specific that was holding them back. A habit they didn't know was a problem. A nutritional gap they didn't realize existed. Small things that made a big difference once we fixed them.

I wanted to gather all of that information in one place. Let me say it again because it's important. This is not medical advice. I'm a trainer, not a doctor. Anything related to your medication, your dosing, your health conditions, that's between you and your healthcare provider. Always consult your doctor before making any changes to your treatment plan. What I'm offering here are practical, evidence-based strategies for the lifestyle piece. The nutrition, the movement, the daily habits that can help you get the most out of your medication. These are things you can actually do, starting today, that might make a real difference. But they work alongside medical care, not instead of it.

If you're reading this, you're probably frustrated. Maybe you started your medication with high hopes and the results just haven't been what you expected. Maybe you lost weight at first but now you're stuck. Maybe you're watching other people succeed and wondering what you're missing.

I want you to know that you're not alone in feeling that way. And you're definitely not broken. There are real reasons why people respond differently to these medications. And there are real things you can do about it.

So let's figure this out together.

How to Use This Book

I've organized this book kind of like a troubleshooting guide. If your medication is working well and you're seeing steady progress, you might not need most of what's in here. But if you're a slow responder, if you've hit a plateau, or if your results just aren't matching your expectations, this book should help you figure out why.

Here's how it's laid out:

Part One covers the basics of GLP-1 medications. What they actually are, how they work in your body, and why people respond so differently. If you're fairly new to these medications, this is a good place to start.

Part Two goes into the fundamentals that most people get wrong. Things like calorie deficits, protein intake, and exercise. For most readers, these chapters are going to be the most valuable. They cover the most common reasons people don't see the results they're hoping for.

Part Three is about more advanced troubleshooting. We'll look at metabolic issues, hormones, lifestyle factors, and some of the deeper things that can affect your progress. If you've tried the basics and they haven't solved your problem, this section should help.

Part Four covers some special situations. Things like losing those last ten or twenty pounds, dealing with weight regain even while you're still on the medication, and considerations for specific groups like older adults or people with conditions like PCOS.

Part Five brings everything together. You'll find practical protocols you can follow and strategies for long-term success.

You don't have to read this book straight through from beginning to end. Feel free to jump to whatever chapter addresses your specific situation. There's also a troubleshooting flowchart in Chapter 14 if you're not sure where to start.

One more thing. This book assumes you're already working with a healthcare provider who prescribed your medication. I'm not going to tell you to change your dose, switch medications, or stop taking anything. Those decisions need to happen between you and your doctor. What I will help you with is optimizing everything else. What you eat, how you move, the habits you build around the medication.

Those are things you have control over, and they matter more than most people realize.

Let's figure out what's been holding you back and get you moving in the right direction.

David Brant,
Vancouver, British Columbia, Canada

PART 1

Understanding GLP-1s

Chapter 1
The GLP-1 Revolution

If you had told me ten years ago that one of the biggest breakthroughs in weight loss would come from studying the saliva of a Gila monster, I probably would have laughed. But that's exactly what happened. And understanding how we got here helps explain why these medications are such a big deal.

What Are GLP-1 Receptor Agonists?

Let's start with the basics. GLP-1, short for glucagon-like peptide-1, is a natural intestinal hormone your body releases after meals. Think of it as a messenger that handles several jobs at once. It prompts your pancreas to produce insulin when blood sugar climbs. It slows down digestion so food doesn't rush through your system. And it tells your brain that you've had enough to eat.

In a healthy person, this hormone does its work quickly and then disappears. Your body breaks it down within minutes using specific enzymes. It's efficient but short-lived.

GLP-1 receptor agonists are medications designed to mimic this natural hormone, but with one key difference. They last much longer. Instead of vanishing in minutes, they keep working for hours or even days. That extended action is what makes them so effective for appetite control and blood sugar management.

The "agonist" part just means they activate the same receptors your natural GLP-1 would use. They're speaking the same language to your body, just with a longer, louder message.

A Brief History: From Gila Monster Venom to Ozempic

Here's where the story gets interesting. During the 1990s, scientists examining Gila monster venom identified a peptide called exendin-4 that resembled human GLP-1. This became the blueprint for the first generation of GLP-1 medications.

Why would a desert lizard produce something like this? Gila monsters eat infrequently, sometimes just a few times per year, so their metabolism needs to be incredibly efficient when they do feed. That same efficiency turned out to have applications for human blood sugar control.

The first medication based on this discovery, exenatide (brand name Byetta), reached the market in 2005 for type 2 diabetes. Patients had to inject it twice daily, which wasn't ideal. But doctors started noticing an unexpected benefit. Their patients were losing weight, and not just a few pounds.

This side effect became impossible to ignore.

The Evolution: Exenatide to Liraglutide to Semaglutide to Tirzepatide

Each new generation of these medications brought meaningful improvements to how patients experienced treatment.

Liraglutide arrived in 2010 as Victoza for diabetes management, requiring just one daily injection instead of two. By 2014, a higher-dose version called Saxenda earned approval specifically for weight management. Patients saw results, though the daily injections and side effects remained challenges for some people.

The real turning point came in 2017 with semaglutide. Marketed as Ozempic for diabetes and later as Wegovy for weight loss, it only required weekly injections. More importantly, it worked better. Clinical trials showed participants losing an average of 15% of their body weight. For someone weighing 200 pounds, that meant 30 pounds gone. Suddenly, everyone was paying attention.

Then tirzepatide entered the scene in 2022 under the names Mounjaro and Zepbound. This medication took a different approach by mimicking two hormones instead of one. It activates both GLP-1 and GIP (glucose-dependent insulinotropic polypeptide) receptors. In trials, participants saw even better results, with average weight loss around

20% of body weight. That level of effectiveness moved the conversation into new territory.

What changed with each generation wasn't just convenience. The patient experience evolved. Fewer injections meant better adherence. Stronger effects meant more dramatic results. And as the medications improved, more people started viewing them as legitimate long-term tools rather than just diabetes drugs with weight loss as an afterthought.

How They Work: The Science of Appetite Suppression and Metabolic Effects

So what's actually happening in your body when you take these medications?

The most noticeable effect is how these drugs quiet the brain's hunger circuits, mainly in the hypothalamus and brainstem. These regions control when you feel hungry and when you feel satisfied. When the medication activates GLP-1 receptors there, appetite signals fade and fullness lasts longer.

For many people, this shift feels profound. They've spent years fighting constant hunger and cravings. Then they start the medication and the internal noise simply quiets. Hours pass without thinking about food. Smaller portions feel satisfying. The mental energy previously spent resisting cravings just evaporates.

Beyond appetite, these medications slow gastric emptying. Food lingers in your stomach longer after you eat, which reinforces that feeling of fullness and helps prevent blood sugar from spiking sharply after meals.

The metabolic effects matter too. These medications improve how your body responds to insulin, leading to better blood sugar control. For people with type 2 diabetes, this benefit is obvious. But even without diabetes, improved insulin sensitivity supports weight loss and overall metabolic health.

Emerging research also suggests these medications may reduce inflammation and improve how your body processes fats, though scientists are still working to understand these effects fully.

Beyond Weight Loss: Cardiovascular, Kidney, and Other Benefits

Here's something that deserves more attention. These medications offer benefits that extend well beyond the number on your scale.

The cardiovascular benefits have been striking. Major studies, including trials published in the New England Journal of Medicine, have demonstrated that semaglutide and similar medications reduce the risk of heart attacks, strokes, and cardiovascular death by approximately 20% in people with existing heart disease. That's a meaningful reduction in life-threatening events.

Even for people without diagnosed heart disease, these

medications tend to improve cardiovascular markers. Blood pressure drops. Cholesterol profiles shift in favorable directions. Inflammation markers decrease throughout the body.

Kidney health shows improvement too, particularly for people with diabetes. Research has demonstrated that GLP-1 medications can slow kidney disease progression, which matters enormously for people already facing kidney challenges.

Scientists are also exploring potential benefits for conditions like fatty liver disease and sleep apnea. Some research is even examining whether these medications might help with Alzheimer's disease and Parkinson's disease, though this work remains in early stages.

And here's something unexpected that keeps coming up. People report changes in other compulsive behaviors. Some say their interest in alcohol decreases. Others notice reduced impulses around shopping or other habits. The brain pathways these medications affect overlap with reward and addiction circuits, which could explain these observations. But this area needs much more study before we draw firm conclusions.

The Current Landscape: Who's Using Them and Why

Millions of people worldwide are now using GLP-1 medications, and that number has grown rapidly over just the past few years.

Many users have type 2 diabetes and take these medications primarily for blood sugar control, which is what they were originally designed to do. But increasingly, people without diabetes are using them specifically for weight management.

The typical weight loss user is someone who has tried other approaches without lasting success. They've followed various diets, joined gyms, worked with nutritionists. Some have lost significant weight multiple times only to regain it. For these people, GLP-1 medications offer something fundamentally different: a tool that addresses the biological drive to eat, not just willpower or discipline.

But the user base is broader than that. Some people take lower doses for modest weight loss or maintenance. Others use them to manage conditions like polycystic ovary syndrome or insulin resistance. And yes, some use them primarily for appearance, which has sparked considerable debate.

Access remains challenging. Shortages have been common. The medications cost over $1,000 monthly without insurance coverage. Insurance policies vary wildly, with some covering them for diabetes but not weight loss, and others refusing coverage entirely. This inconsistency has driven growth in compounding pharmacies making their own versions, raising separate questions about safety and regulation.

A broader cultural conversation is happening too. Some view these medications as miraculous. Others worry about overprescription or enabling people to avoid necessary lifestyle changes. Concerns about long-term safety persist since widespread use is relatively new. Questions about what happens when people stop taking them remain partially unanswered.

All of these concerns deserve consideration. But here's what I've observed working with real people. For many, these medications have been genuinely transformative. They've accomplished things that previously felt impossible. Their health markers have moved into healthier ranges. They feel better physically and emotionally.

At the same time, medication alone isn't enough. The people who achieve the best results treat it as one tool among several. They prioritize nutrition. They stay physically active. They work on their relationship with food and eating. The medication provides an advantage, but success still requires consistent effort.

That's what the rest of this book addresses. How to do that work effectively so the medication can deliver the results you're hoping for.

Chapter 2
Why Some People Don't Respond as Expected

A few months ago, a client came into my gym looking completely deflated. She'd been on semaglutide for twelve weeks and had lost eight pounds. Eight pounds. She should have been celebrating, but instead she was ready to quit. Why? Because her sister had lost twenty-five pounds in the same timeframe on the same medication.

This happens all the time. Someone starts a GLP-1 medication with high expectations, often based on what they've seen other people achieve. Then their own experience doesn't match up, and they feel like something must be wrong with them. But here's what I've learned. Response to these medications varies wildly from person to person. Understanding why that happens can save you a lot of frustration.

What Does "Responding" Actually Mean?

Before we talk about why some people don't respond well, we need to define what a good response actually looks like. This is where a lot of confusion starts.

In clinical trials, researchers typically consider a medication effective if someone loses 5% or more of their body weight. For a person weighing 200 pounds, that's just 10 pounds. Now, I know what you're thinking. Ten pounds doesn't sound like much, especially when you're hearing stories about people losing fifty or sixty pounds.

But from a medical perspective, even modest weight loss can produce significant health benefits. Blood pressure improves. Blood sugar control gets better. Inflammation decreases. A 5% weight loss can be genuinely meaningful for your health, even if it doesn't feel dramatic.

The challenge is that most people aren't taking these medications just for a 5% reduction. They want substantial weight loss. They're thinking 15%, 20%, maybe more. And the success stories they see online and hear from friends set those expectations even higher.

So when we talk about responding to the medication, we need to separate clinical response from personal goals. You might be responding perfectly well from a medical standpoint while still feeling disappointed because your results don't match what you were hoping for.

Realistic expectations for most people taking GLP-1

medications look something like this. In the first three to six months, you might lose 10-15% of your body weight if you're on a therapeutic dose and following good nutrition habits. Some people will lose more. Some will lose less. After that initial period, weight loss typically slows down. You might continue losing, but at a slower pace. By the one-year mark, average weight loss ranges from 15-20% depending on the specific medication and dose.

But averages don't tell individual stories. Some people lose 30% of their body weight. Others lose 5%. Both are responding to the medication, just differently.

The Spectrum of Response: Non-Responders vs. Slow Responders vs. Plateaus

Not everyone's journey with these medications follows the same path. Let me break down the different experiences people have.

True non-responders are people who see little to no weight loss despite being on an adequate dose for several months. We're talking less than 5% weight loss after six months. This group exists, but it's smaller than you might think. Estimates suggest around 10-15% of people fall into this category. If you're in this group, the medication simply isn't doing much for your appetite or metabolism, even though you're taking it correctly.

Slow responders are much more common. These are people

who do lose weight, but at a pace that feels frustratingly slow compared to what they expected. Maybe they lose one pound every two weeks instead of two pounds per week. Maybe they drop 8% of their body weight when they were hoping for 15%. The medication is working, but not as dramatically as they'd hoped. This describes a significant portion of GLP-1 users.

Then there are people who have a great initial response but hit a plateau. They might lose twenty pounds in the first three months and then nothing for the next two months. The weight loss just stops, even though they're still taking the medication and haven't changed their habits. Plateaus are incredibly common and can happen at any point in the process.

It's important to understand that these aren't permanent categories. A slow responder might pick up speed with some adjustments. Someone who plateaus might start losing again once they troubleshoot what's holding them back. And even true non-responders sometimes find success by switching medications or addressing underlying issues that were interfering with their response.

The key is figuring out which category you're in and why. That's what the rest of this book is designed to help you do.

Individual Variation: Genetics, Metabolism, and Biological Factors

So why do people respond so differently? The honest

answer is that we don't fully understand all the reasons yet. But we do know several factors that play a role.

Genetics matter. Research has identified genetic variations that affect how people respond to GLP-1 medications. Some people have versions of certain genes that make them more or less sensitive to these drugs. Your genetic makeup influences things like how quickly your body breaks down the medication, how strongly it activates receptors in your brain and gut, and how your metabolism responds overall.

You can't change your genetics, obviously. But understanding that genetic differences exist can help you stop blaming yourself if your response isn't what you expected.

Baseline metabolism varies enormously between people. Some people naturally burn more calories at rest. Others have slower metabolic rates. Your metabolic rate depends on factors like muscle mass, thyroid function, age, and hormonal balance. Two people of the same height and weight can have metabolic rates that differ by several hundred calories per day. That difference adds up over time and affects weight loss speed.

Insulin resistance is another big factor. People with significant insulin resistance often have a harder time losing weight, even on GLP-1 medications. The medication helps improve insulin sensitivity, which is great. But if you're starting from a place of severe insulin resistance, progress might be slower than for someone with better metabolic health to begin with.

Your gut microbiome probably plays a role too. Emerging research suggests that the bacteria living in your digestive system influence how you respond to various interventions, including medications. Some bacterial profiles seem to support weight loss better than others. This field is still developing, but it's clear that gut health matters.

Age affects response as well. Older adults tend to lose weight more slowly than younger people, partly because metabolism naturally slows with age and partly because hormonal changes make fat loss more challenging. This doesn't mean older people can't succeed on these medications. They absolutely can. But expectations might need to adjust.

And then there's your weight loss history. If you've lost and regained weight multiple times over the years, your body may have adapted in ways that make subsequent weight loss harder. Repeated dieting can lower your metabolic rate and change how your body regulates hunger hormones. This adaptive response is sometimes called metabolic adaptation, and it can dampen your response to GLP-1 medications.

Common Misconceptions About How GLP-1s Work

Let me clear up some misunderstandings that often trip people up.

Misconception number one is that the medication does all the work. A lot of people think that once they start the injection, weight loss will happen automatically. They believe the medication will override everything else and the pounds will just melt off. That's not how it works. The medication suppresses appetite, which makes it easier to eat less. But you still need to actually eat less. You still need to make decent food choices. You still need to move your body. The medication is a powerful tool, but it's not magic.

Misconception number two is that everyone responds the same way. We've already covered this, but it's worth repeating. Individual responses vary dramatically. Just because your friend lost thirty pounds doesn't mean you will. Comparing yourself to others will only make you miserable.

Misconception number three is that more medication equals more weight loss. Some people assume that if they're not losing weight fast enough, they just need a higher dose. Sometimes that's true. But often the issue isn't the dose. It's something else entirely, like not being in a calorie deficit or not getting enough protein or not moving enough. Increasing the dose won't fix those problems. It might just give you worse side effects.

Misconception number four is that weight loss will be steady and linear. In reality, weight loss is messy. You might lose three pounds one week, nothing the next week, gain a pound the following week, then drop two pounds after that. Water retention, hormones, digestion, and dozens of other factors cause daily and weekly fluctuations. What matters is the trend over several weeks and months, not what happens day to day.

Misconception number five is that once you start losing weight, it will continue indefinitely. Your body doesn't work that way. As you lose weight, your body adapts. Your metabolism slows down slightly because you have less body mass to maintain. Your hunger hormones shift. Your body becomes more efficient at conserving energy. All of these adaptations mean that weight loss naturally slows over time. Plateaus aren't failures. They're normal physiological responses.

The 10-20% Who Don't See Dramatic Results: You're Not Alone

If you're reading this book, there's a decent chance you fall into this group. Maybe you've been on a GLP-1 medication for several months and your results have been underwhelming. Maybe you lost some weight initially but nothing dramatic. Maybe you've hit a frustrating plateau that won't budge.

First, I want you to know that you're not alone. Despite what social media might make you think, not everyone is losing fifty pounds on these medications. A significant minority of people don't get dramatic results, at least not without making additional changes beyond just taking the medication.

This doesn't mean you're broken. It doesn't mean you're doing something wrong. And it definitely doesn't mean you should give up.

What it usually means is that there are specific factors interfering with your response. Maybe you're not in as deep a calorie deficit as you think. Maybe your protein intake is too low and you're losing muscle along with fat. Maybe stress or poor sleep is affecting your hormones in ways that slow progress. Maybe there's an underlying metabolic issue that needs addressing.

The good news is that most of these factors are identifiable and fixable. That's what the next several chapters are all about. We're going to walk through the most common reasons people don't see the results they want, and more importantly, what you can do about each one.

Understanding That Medication Is Only One Piece of the Puzzle

Here's the bottom line. GLP-1 medications are incredibly powerful. They've helped millions of people lose weight and improve their health. But they work best when combined with good nutrition, regular movement, adequate sleep, stress management, and sustainable habits.

Think of the medication as a tool that makes those other things easier. It quiets your appetite so eating less doesn't feel like torture. It helps regulate your blood sugar so you have more stable energy. It takes away some of the constant mental noise around food. Those advantages are huge.

But the medication can't force you into a calorie deficit. It can't make you eat enough protein. It can't make you move your body. It can't fix poor sleep or chronic stress. Those pieces are still up to you.

The people who get the best results are the ones who use the medication as a foundation and then build everything else on top of it. They track their food, at least loosely, to make sure they're actually in a deficit. They prioritize protein to protect their muscle. They exercise consistently. They work on their habits and their relationship with food.

That might sound like a lot of work. And honestly, it is some work. But it's so much less work than trying to do all of those things without the medication. The medication gives you a significant advantage. It takes willpower and hunger out of the equation to a large degree. But it doesn't eliminate the need for the other fundamentals.

If your results so far haven't been what you hoped for, don't give up. Instead, let's figure out what's been holding you back. In the next chapter, we'll start with the single biggest issue I see: people who think they're eating in a deficit but actually aren't.

The Fundamentals (What Most People Get Wrong)

Chapter 3
Understanding Energy Balance (Without the Guilt)

You've probably heard your entire life to "just eat less." Maybe from doctors, maybe from well-meaning friends, maybe from diet culture screaming at you from every direction. And honestly, that advice has probably made you feel terrible. Like weight loss is simply a matter of willpower, and if you're struggling, it's because you're not trying hard enough.

Here's the truth. Your body is a complicated mechanism. Your thyroid function, conditions like PCOS, your genetics, your metabolism, your hormone levels, your sleep quality, even certain medications you take. All of these factors influence how your body processes food and how easily you lose or gain weight. For some people, these factors play a huge role in why weight loss feels nearly impossible.

So no, it's not as simple as "just eat less." Your body is more complex than that, and your struggle is real and valid.

Having said that, we do need to take an honest look at

energy balance. Not because it's the only thing that matters. Not because everything else can be ignored. But because understanding the relationship between the energy you take in and the energy your body uses is one piece of the puzzle. And for a lot of people on GLP-1 medications who aren't seeing the results they hoped for, this piece is where they're getting stuck.

This chapter isn't about judgment or restriction. It's about understanding what might be happening so you can make informed choices about what to adjust.

Why Energy Balance Matters Even When Other Factors Are at Play

Let me start by acknowledging something important. Energy balance isn't the only thing that affects weight loss. Not even close.

If you have a thyroid condition, your metabolism might be running slower than average. If you have PCOS, your body might handle insulin differently in ways that make fat storage easier and fat loss harder. If you've been on certain medications like antidepressants or steroids, those can affect your weight too. Genetics play a role in how efficiently your body uses energy. Some people just naturally have slower metabolisms than others.

All of that is real, and it matters. If you suspect something like this might be affecting you, it's absolutely worth talking to your doctor and getting tested. Addressing underlying medical issues can make a real difference.

But here's the thing. Even with all of those factors, energy balance still matters. It's not the only piece of the puzzle, but it is a piece. Your body still needs a certain amount of energy to function, and if you're consistently taking in more than that amount, weight loss won't happen, even on GLP-1 medications.

Think of it this way. Medical conditions and metabolic factors affect how much energy your body needs. They change the equation. But they don't eliminate the equation entirely. You might need to eat less than the average person your size to lose weight, which isn't fair. But identifying that gap is still important.

So yes, there are many factors at play. We'll talk about several of them in later chapters. But right now, we're focusing on energy balance because it's one of the most common places people get stuck, and it's something you can actually do something about.

Understanding How Much Energy Your Body Actually Needs

Here's something that surprises a lot of people. Your body's energy needs are probably lower than you think, especially if you've already lost some weight or if you're not very active.

Let me give you a practical example. Let's say you're a

45-year-old woman who's 5'5" and weighs 180 pounds. Before starting a GLP-1 medication, you might have been eating around 2,500 or even 3,000 calories per day. That's what it took to maintain your weight at that activity level.

Now you start the medication. Your appetite drops. You're eating much less than before. Let's say you're down to around 2,000 calories per day. That feels like a massive reduction. You're eating way less than you used to. But here's the thing. For someone your size with a moderate activity level, your body might only need about 1,800 to 2,000 calories per day to maintain your current weight.

So even though you've cut your intake significantly, you might only be in a very small deficit, or possibly no deficit at all. The weight loss will be slow or nonexistent, even though you genuinely are eating much less than before.

Or let's say you're a 50-year-old man who's 5'10" and weighs 220 pounds. You were probably eating 3,000 to 3,500 calories per day to maintain that weight. You start your GLP-1 medication and drop down to 2,500 calories per day. That's a huge reduction, and you should feel proud of that change. But your body at that weight and activity level might need around 2,400 to 2,600 calories per day to maintain. You're barely in a deficit, which means weight loss will be very slow.

The math changes as you lose weight too. If that woman drops from 180 pounds to 160 pounds, her body now needs fewer calories to function because there's less of her to maintain. What was a deficit at 180 pounds might not be a deficit anymore at 160 pounds.

So how do you figure out how much your body actually needs? There are calculators online that estimate your Total Daily Energy Expenditure, or TDEE. You enter your age, sex, height, weight, and activity level, and it gives you an estimate. These aren't perfect, but they're a reasonable starting point.

For women, a rough estimate is:
- Sedentary (little to no exercise): 12-14 calories per pound of body weight
- Lightly active (light exercise 1-3 days per week): 14-16 calories per pound
- Moderately active (moderate exercise 3-5 days per week): 16-18 calories per pound

For men, estimates are typically:
- Sedentary: 14-16 calories per pound of body weight
- Lightly active: 16-18 calories per pound
- Moderately active: 18-20 calories per pound

These are rough guidelines. Your actual needs might be higher or lower depending on your metabolism, muscle mass, and other factors. But they give you a ballpark.

To lose weight, you generally need to eat less than your TDEE. A deficit of 300 to 500 calories per day typically results in steady weight loss of about half a pound to one pound per week. Larger deficits can work too, but they're harder to sustain and can lead to muscle loss if you're not careful.

The point isn't to make you obsess over these numbers. The point is to help you understand that even though you're eating way less than before, you might not be eating less than your body currently needs. That's not a failure. It's just information that helps you figure out your next step.

The Common Assumption: Appetite Suppression Equals Automatic Weight Loss

This is one of the most common misconceptions I see. People start their GLP-1 medication, their appetite drops, they're eating less than they used to, and they assume the weight will just come off automatically.

For some people, that's exactly what happens. Their appetite drops so dramatically that they naturally end up in a significant calorie deficit without trying. They lose weight steadily and everything works great.

But for a lot of people, it doesn't work out that way. Their appetite decreases, sure. They're eating smaller portions. They're not snacking as much. But they're still eating enough that weight loss is slow or nonexistent.

Why does this happen? A few reasons.

First, appetite suppression varies in intensity. Some people lose almost all interest in food. Others just feel less hungry than before but still have a normal appetite. If your appetite suppression is on the milder end, you might still be eating at or near your maintenance calories without realizing it.

Second, people adjust their eating in ways that compensate for reduced appetite. Maybe you're not hungry for breakfast anymore, so you skip it. Great. But then at dinner, you eat a larger portion because you have room for it. Or you're not snacking during the day, but you're having dessert at night. The total amount you're eating might not have changed as much as you think.

Third, reduced appetite doesn't prevent you from eating when food is available, especially if it's really good food or you're in a social setting. Your hunger might be lower, but you can still eat a full meal at a restaurant or finish what's on your plate at a family dinner.

None of this means you're doing anything wrong. It just means that appetite suppression alone doesn't guarantee you're in the deficit needed for weight loss.

Why You Might Not Be in a Deficit Even Though You're Eating Less

Let's talk about why eating less than you used to doesn't necessarily mean you're in a deficit.

Your body's energy needs change as you lose weight. As you get smaller, you require less energy to function because there's less of you to maintain. This is completely normal.

Here's a practical example. Let's say you weigh 200 pounds and your body needs about 2,200 calories per day to maintain that weight. You start a GLP-1 medication and begin eating 1,800 calories per day. That's a 400-calorie deficit. You lose weight steadily for a few months.

But now you weigh 180 pounds. At this lower weight, your body only needs about 2,000 calories per day to maintain. If you're still eating 1,800 calories, your deficit has shrunk to just 200 calories per day. Weight loss will be much slower. And if your activity level has decreased at all, which often happens, you might not be in a deficit anymore.

This isn't your fault. This is just how bodies work. But it explains why eating the same amount that worked initially might stop producing results over time.

There's also the issue of metabolic adaptation. When you lose weight, especially if you lose it quickly, your metabolism can slow down beyond what you'd expect from weight loss alone. Your body becomes more efficient at using energy. It tries to conserve. This adaptation is your body's way of protecting against what it perceives as a threat.

This isn't a character flaw or a sign that you broke your metabolism. It's a normal physiological response. But it does mean that creating and maintaining a deficit can be harder than the basic math suggests.

Understanding the "I'm Barely Eating" Paradox:
Calorie-Dense Foods in Small Portions

One of the trickiest things about eating on GLP-1 medications is that you can genuinely feel like you're barely eating while still consuming quite a bit of energy.

Here's how this happens. The medication suppresses your appetite, so you can only handle small portions. You might eat a quarter of what you used to eat at a meal. That feels like nothing. But if that small portion is calorie-dense, you're still taking in significant energy.

Let me give you some real examples from clients I've worked with.

One woman was having a small bowl of granola with whole milk for breakfast. The portion looked tiny to her, maybe half a cup of granola and a splash of milk. She felt like she was barely eating. But that small bowl had about 400 calories. For someone trying to lose weight on 1,500 calories a day, that's more than a quarter of her daily intake in what felt like a snack-sized portion.

Another client would have a few pieces of cheese and some crackers in the afternoon. Maybe five or six crackers and a couple ounces of cheese. It didn't feel like much food at all. But it was easily 300 calories. He was doing this most days without thinking about it because the portion seemed so small.

These aren't bad foods. Granola, cheese, and crackers are

all fine. But they're calorie-dense, meaning they pack a lot of energy into a small volume. When your appetite is suppressed and you can only eat small amounts, it's really easy to choose calorie-dense foods because they're more satisfying in small quantities.

The problem is that your stomach might feel satisfied, but you haven't created much of a deficit.

Other common calorie-dense foods that trip people up include nuts, nut butters, oils and butter, avocados, dried fruit, chocolate, and baked goods. Even in small amounts, these foods contribute significant calories. A tablespoon of peanut butter is about 100 calories. A small handful of almonds is 150 calories. A drizzle of olive oil is 120 calories.

None of this means you shouldn't eat these foods. But it does mean you need to be aware of how they fit into your overall intake, especially when you're eating small portions that don't feel like much.

Liquid Calories: Coffee Drinks, Alcohol, and Smoothies That Can Stall Progress

Liquid calories are another huge blind spot for people on GLP-1 medications.

When your appetite is suppressed, you might not feel like eating much solid food. But drinking doesn't trigger the same fullness signals. You can consume hundreds of calories in beverages without feeling like you've eaten anything at all.

Coffee drinks are a major culprit. A plain black coffee has almost no calories. But add cream, sugar, flavored syrup, or make it a latte or cappuccino, and you're looking at 200 to 500 calories depending on the size and ingredients. If you're having one or two of these per day, that's a significant portion of your energy intake.

I worked with a client who couldn't figure out why she wasn't losing weight. She was eating very little, maybe one small meal per day. But she was having three large iced coffees with cream and sugar throughout the day. Each one had about 300 calories. That's 900 calories just from coffee. She'd essentially replaced food with caloric beverages without realizing it.

Alcohol is another big one. Alcohol contains seven calories per gram, almost as much as fat. A glass of wine has about 120 to 150 calories. A beer has 150 to 200 calories. Mixed drinks can be even higher, especially if they contain juice or sugary mixers. If you're having a couple of drinks most evenings, that can easily be 300 to 500 calories that don't register as eating.

Smoothies seem healthy, and they can be. But they can also pack in a surprising number of calories. Fruit, yogurt, protein powder, nut butter, juice, milk. A large smoothie can easily hit 400 to 600 calories. If you're drinking it instead of eating a meal, that might be fine. But if it's in addition to your meals, or if you're having multiple smoothies per day, the calories add up quickly.

Juice, soda, sweet tea, energy drinks, and even some protein shakes can contribute hundreds of calories without providing much satiety. Your body doesn't register liquid calories the same way it registers solid food, so you don't feel fuller after drinking them.

The tricky part is that GLP-1 medications reduce your hunger for food, but they don't necessarily reduce your desire for beverages. You might not want to eat, but you still want your morning latte or evening glass of wine. Those habits can persist even when your eating habits change dramatically.

Weekend Eating Patterns: How Two Days Can Shift Your Weekly Balance

This one surprises people. You can be really consistent with your eating Monday through Friday, creating a nice deficit, and then undo a lot of that progress over the weekend without even realizing it.

Here's how the math works. Let's say you're aiming for a 500-calorie deficit per day to lose about one pound per week. Monday through Friday, you stick to your plan. That's a 2,500-calorie deficit for the week. Great.

But then Saturday comes. You sleep in, you have a big brunch with friends. Pancakes, bacon, maybe a mimosa. Then in the evening, you go out for dinner and have a few drinks. You're not going crazy, but you're definitely eating and drinking more than usual. Between brunch, dinner, drinks, and some snacking, you end up eating 1,000 calories over your target for the day.

Sunday, you're a bit more relaxed too. Maybe not as much as Saturday, but you have a larger breakfast, you have dessert after dinner, you snack while watching TV. You end up 500 calories over your target.

That's 1,500 calories over your target for the weekend. Your weekly deficit of 2,500 calories just became a 1,000-calorie deficit. Instead of losing one pound that week, you'll lose less than half a pound. And if your weekends are consistently like this, your progress will be much slower than expected.

The frustrating part is that weekday eating feels like your normal, and weekend eating feels like just a little relaxation. But those two days represent almost 30% of your week. They have a significant impact on your overall energy balance.

This pattern is really common. People are structured and disciplined during the work week. Then the weekend hits and routines go out the window. Social events, dining out, sleeping in and skipping breakfast then having a huge lunch, having a few drinks, grabbing takeout. None of it feels excessive in the moment, but it adds up.

GLP-1 medications help with this to some degree. Your appetite is lower even on weekends, so you might naturally eat less at that brunch or dinner. But appetite suppression doesn't prevent you from eating when food is in front of you, especially if it's really good food or if you're in a social setting where everyone else is eating.

How to Track Without Obsession: Practical Calorie Awareness

Okay, so energy balance matters. But I'm not suggesting you need to weigh every morsel of food and log it in an app for the rest of your life. That's not sustainable, and for some people, it can trigger unhealthy behaviors around food.

What I am suggesting is developing some level of awareness. You need a general sense of how much energy you're taking in and whether it's in line with your body's needs and your goals.

For some people, loose tracking works well. You don't measure everything precisely, but you have a rough idea of portion sizes and calorie content. You might log your food a few days per week just to check in, or you might estimate in your head. This approach gives you enough information to stay on track without becoming obsessive.

For others, more precise tracking is helpful, at least initially. Using a free app like Lose It, MyFitnessPal, or Cronometer for a few weeks can be really educational. You learn what appropriate portions look like. You discover which foods are more calorie-dense than you realized. You become aware of patterns in your eating. Once you have that knowledge, you can often back off the detailed tracking and maintain awareness without it.

Some people do better with no formal tracking at all. Instead, they focus on practical strategies like eating mostly whole foods, having protein at every meal, limiting calorie-dense foods, and paying attention to hunger and fullness cues. If this approach works for you and you're getting results, that's great. But if you're not seeing progress, some level of tracking might help you identify the issue.

The key is finding an approach that gives you useful information without making you miserable or anxious. Tracking should be a tool, not a source of stress.

Mindful Awareness vs. Rigid Tracking: Finding What Works for You

There's a spectrum between completely ignoring calories and obsessively tracking every single thing you eat. Most people do best somewhere in the middle.

Mindful awareness means paying attention to what and how much you're eating without necessarily quantifying everything. You notice portion sizes. You think about whether you're actually hungry or just eating out of habit. You're conscious of higher-calorie foods and make intentional choices about when to include them. You check in with yourself about how your eating aligns with your goals.

This approach works well for people who have a decent baseline understanding of nutrition and portion sizes. It also works for people who find that detailed tracking makes them anxious or triggers unhealthy thought patterns.

Rigid tracking means measuring and logging everything you eat, hitting specific calorie targets every day, and monitoring your intake closely. This approach provides the most data and can be really effective for people who like structure and want precise control over their results.

But rigid tracking has downsides. It can be time-consuming. It can make eating feel like a chore. For some people, it creates an unhealthy relationship with food where nothing feels okay to eat unless it fits the numbers perfectly. And it can be hard to sustain long-term.

Most people benefit from starting with some tracking to build awareness, then gradually loosening up as they develop better intuition about portion sizes and food choices. You might track closely for a month to learn, then switch to tracking a few days per week, then eventually just check in occasionally when you feel like you might be drifting off track.

The right approach is the one you can actually stick with. If tracking every day makes you crazy, don't do it. Find a looser method that still gives you enough information. If you're the type of person who likes data and structure, tracking might work great for you. There's no one right way.

Action Steps: Simple Tracking Methods for Beginners

Let me give you some practical ways to develop better awareness of your energy balance without making it your full-time job.

Start by tracking for just one week. Don't change anything about how you're eating. Just log everything as accurately as you can. This gives you a baseline. You'll see how much you're actually eating, where most of your calories are coming from, and whether you have patterns you weren't aware of. After that week, you can decide if you want to keep tracking or if you have enough information.

Focus on the big contributors first. Instead of worrying about every little thing, pay attention to the foods and meals that contribute the most calories. For most people, that's beverages, snacks, oils and fats used in cooking, and restaurant meals. If you can get a handle on those, you've addressed the majority of your intake without obsessing over every bite.

Invest in a digital scale. Learn portion sizes for your most common foods. You don't need to weigh food forever. But weighing and measuring for a week or two teaches you what portions actually look like. Once you know that a serving of rice is about the size of your fist or that a tablespoon of peanut butter is smaller than you thought, you can eyeball portions more accurately going forward.

Use the hand method for rough estimates. Your palm is about one serving of protein. Your fist is about one serving of vegetables or carbs. Your thumb is about one serving of fats. This isn't precise, but it gives you a framework for building balanced meals without measuring.

Check in regularly without obsessing. You might track

your food one day per week just to make sure you're still on track. Or you might do a three-day food log once per month. Regular check-ins help you catch drift before it becomes a problem, without requiring constant monitoring.

Pay attention to patterns, not perfection. If you notice you're consistently going over your needs on weekends, that's useful information. If you see that your coffee drinks are contributing more calories than you realized, you can make an adjustment. The goal is awareness and gentle course correction, not hitting perfect numbers every single day.

Remember, the GLP-1 medication is doing a lot of heavy lifting here. It's making it easier to eat less without feeling deprived. You're just adding some awareness on top of that advantage to make sure you're actually creating the deficit you need. That's not restrictive or obsessive. That's just being intentional about your goals.

Energy balance isn't the only thing that matters for weight loss on GLP-1 medications. But it's a foundational piece. If this piece isn't in place, the other strategies we'll talk about in upcoming chapters won't help as much as they should. Get your energy balance sorted, and everything else becomes easier.

Chapter 4
Protein: The Non-Negotiable

A few months ago, a client came in celebrating. She'd lost thirty pounds on semaglutide and felt amazing. Her clothes fit better, her energy was up, and she was thrilled with her progress. Then we did a body composition scan. She'd lost thirty pounds, but twelve of those pounds were muscle. Almost 40% of her weight loss wasn't fat. It was the tissue that keeps her metabolism running, her bones strong, and her body functional.

She was devastated. And honestly, I felt terrible for not catching it sooner. But here's the thing. This is incredibly common. When you lose weight rapidly on GLP-1 medications without paying attention to protein, a significant portion of what you lose is muscle. And that matters more than most people realize.

Why Protein Matters Even More on GLP-1s
When you're not on any medication and losing weight

slowly through diet and exercise, you'll naturally lose some muscle along with fat. That's just how weight loss works. But typically, if you're doing things right, about 75-80% of what you lose is fat and 20-25% is muscle. That ratio isn't great, but it's manageable.

On GLP-1 medications, the situation changes. You're losing weight faster than you would through diet and exercise alone. Your appetite is so suppressed that you're eating much less food overall. And when you're eating less food, you're almost certainly eating less protein, unless you're being very intentional about it.

The combination of rapid weight loss and low protein intake creates the perfect storm for muscle loss. I've seen people lose weight at a 50-50 ratio: half fat, half muscle. Some people even worse than that.

Why does this matter? A few reasons.

First, muscle is metabolically active tissue. It burns calories even when you're sitting still. The more muscle you have, the higher your resting metabolic rate. When you lose muscle, your metabolism slows down more than it would from weight loss alone. This makes it easier to regain weight later and harder to continue losing weight as you get closer to your goal.

Second, muscle is what gives your body shape and definition. You can lose a lot of weight and still look soft or undefined if you've lost too much muscle along the way. A lot of people are surprised and disappointed when they hit their goal weight and don't look the way they expected. Often, the issue is that they lost too much muscle during the process.

Third, muscle is functional. It keeps you strong, mobile, and independent. It protects your bones and joints. It helps prevent falls and injuries as you age. Losing muscle isn't just about aesthetics or metabolism. It's about your quality of life.

And fourth, muscle loss can leave you in a tough spot if you ever stop taking the medication. Your metabolism is lower, your muscle mass is depleted, and regaining weight becomes much easier. A lot of people find themselves worse off than when they started if they don't protect their muscle during weight loss.

The good news is that adequate protein intake can dramatically reduce muscle loss. It won't eliminate it entirely, but it can shift that ratio back to something much more favorable. Instead of losing 40% muscle, you might lose 15-20% muscle. That's a huge difference in terms of your metabolism, your body composition, and your long-term success.

Muscle Loss vs. Fat Loss: Protecting Your Metabolism

Let me give you a concrete example of why this matters.

Let's say you weigh 200 pounds and lose 40 pounds over six months on a GLP-1 medication. Congratulations, that's a great accomplishment. But the composition of that weight loss makes all the difference.

Scenario one: You don't prioritize protein. You lose 40 pounds, but 16 of those pounds are muscle. You've lost 24 pounds of fat and 16 pounds of muscle. You now weigh 160 pounds.

Scenario two: You do prioritize protein. You still lose 40 pounds, but only 8 of those pounds are muscle. You've lost 32 pounds of fat and 8 pounds of muscle. You also weigh 160 pounds.

On the scale, these scenarios look identical. But they're dramatically different.

In scenario one, you've lost a significant amount of metabolically active tissue. Your resting metabolic rate has dropped more than it should have just from weight loss. You're weaker. Your body composition isn't as good as it could be. If you stop the medication, regaining weight will be easier because your metabolism is suppressed.

In scenario two, you've preserved much more muscle. Your metabolism hasn't dropped as much. You're stronger. You look more toned and defined. If you stop the medication, you're in a much better position to maintain your weight loss.

The difference between these scenarios often comes down to protein intake. That and resistance training, which we'll talk about in the next chapter. But protein is the foundation. You cannot build or maintain muscle without adequate protein, no matter how much you exercise.

Your body needs protein to repair and maintain muscle

tissue. When you're in a calorie deficit, which you need to be for weight loss, your body is looking for sources of energy. If you're not eating enough protein, your body will break down muscle tissue to get the amino acids it needs. It's easier for your body to cannibalize muscle than to mobilize fat in some situations, especially during rapid weight loss.

Adequate protein intake sends a signal to your body that it has the building blocks it needs. It doesn't have to break down muscle for amino acids. It can preserve that tissue and focus on burning fat instead. It's not perfect protection, but it makes a significant difference.

How Much Protein Do You Actually Need?

This is where people get confused because there's a lot of conflicting information out there.

The official recommendation for protein is 0.8 grams per kilogram of body weight, which works out to about 0.36 grams per pound. For a 180-pound person, that's about 65 grams of protein per day. But here's the thing. That recommendation is designed to prevent deficiency. It's the minimum amount you need to avoid losing muscle if you're sedentary and not trying to lose weight.

When you're trying to lose weight, especially rapidly, you need significantly more protein than that. The research pretty consistently shows that protein intakes of 0.7 to 1.0 grams per pound of your goal body weight are ideal for preserving muscle during weight loss.

So if you currently weigh 200 pounds but your goal weight is 160 pounds, you should aim for 112 to 160 grams of protein per day. That's a wide range, and where you fall in that range depends on a few factors.

If you're doing resistance training regularly, aim for the higher end. If you're older, aim for the higher end because older adults need more protein to maintain muscle. If you're losing weight very rapidly, aim for the higher end. If you're younger, less active, and losing weight more slowly, you can probably get away with the lower end of the range.

A reasonable target for most people is around 0.8 to 1.0 grams per pound of goal body weight. So for that person aiming for 160 pounds, about 130 to 160 grams per day would be a solid goal.

I know that probably sounds like a lot. Especially if you're barely hungry and can only eat small portions. But it's doable, and it's important.

Meeting Protein Goals When You're Never Hungry

This is the challenge. Your appetite is suppressed. You can barely finish a small meal. How are you supposed to eat 130 grams of protein when you're not even hungry?

The key is prioritizing protein at every eating opportunity. When you do eat, protein needs to be the main event, not an afterthought.

Start with protein at every meal. Before you eat anything else, eat your protein source. Chicken, fish, eggs, Greek yogurt, cottage cheese, lean beef, tofu, whatever your protein source is. Eat that first. If you fill up before finishing your meal, at least you got the protein in.

This is a big mindset shift for a lot of people. You might be used to having a balanced plate with vegetables, carbs, and protein all together. But when your appetite is limited, protein has to come first. You can have the other stuff if there's room, but protein is non-negotiable.

Choose protein-dense foods over protein-containing foods. There's a difference. A piece of chicken breast is protein-dense. It's mostly protein with minimal carbs or fat. A bean burrito contains protein, but it also contains a lot of carbs and fat. When you can only eat small amounts, you need foods that pack the most protein into the smallest volume.

Good protein-dense choices include chicken breast, turkey breast, white fish like cod or tilapia, shrimp, eggs, fat-free or low-fat Greek yogurt, cottage cheese, protein powder, and very lean cuts of beef or pork. These foods give you the most protein per bite.

Foods that contain protein but aren't protein-dense include beans, lentils, quinoa, and nuts. These are all healthy foods, but they're not efficient protein sources when your appetite is limited. A cup of black beans has about 15 grams of protein but also 40 grams of carbs. Three ounces of chicken breast has about 26 grams of protein and almost no carbs. When you can only eat small portions, the chicken is a better choice for meeting protein goals.

Spread your protein throughout the day. Your body can only use so much protein at once for muscle building. Eating 100 grams of protein in one meal isn't as effective as spreading 25 to 30 grams across four meals. If you're only eating once or twice a day because of appetite suppression, you're making it harder to meet your protein needs and your body can't use all that protein as efficiently.

Try to eat at least three times a day, even if the meals are small. Each meal should have 25 to 40 grams of protein depending on your total goal. This distribution is better for muscle preservation than eating all your protein at once.

High-Protein Food Strategies and Meal Timing

Let me give you some practical strategies for getting enough protein when you're not hungry.

Make protein shakes your friend. If solid food is hard to get down, liquids are usually easier. A protein shake made with protein powder, milk or a milk alternative, and maybe some fruit can pack 25 to 35 grams of protein into a drink that goes down easily. You can have one in the morning or between meals without feeling overly full.

Use Greek yogurt as a base. Plain, fat-free Greek yogurt has about 15 to 20 grams of protein per cup and it's easy to eat.

Add some berries, a drizzle of honey, maybe a little granola if you have room. It's a protein-rich snack or small meal that doesn't require much appetite.

Keep protein-rich snacks available. Hard-boiled eggs, string cheese, deli turkey, beef jerky, cottage cheese, edamame. These are all portable, easy options when you need to get some protein in but don't want a full meal.

Add protein powder to things. You can mix unflavored or vanilla protein powder into oatmeal, yogurt, pancake batter, soups, or even mashed potatoes. It's a way to boost the protein content of foods you're already eating without adding volume.

Choose fattier proteins if you need more calories. If you're struggling to eat enough overall and protein feels like it's filling you up too much, you can choose fattier cuts of meat or fish. Salmon, for example, has healthy fats and protein. Same with chicken thighs instead of breast. The fat adds calories without adding volume, and you're still getting good protein.

Front-load your protein earlier in the day if you can. A lot of people on GLP-1s find that their appetite is slightly better in the morning and gets worse as the day goes on. If that's you, prioritize getting a big protein hit at breakfast. Eggs, Greek yogurt, a protein shake, whatever works. Get 30 to 40 grams in early, and the rest of the day becomes more manageable.

Plan your meals around protein, not around what sounds good. This is tough because when you're not hungry, nothing sounds good. But instead of asking yourself what you feel like eating, ask yourself what protein source you can tolerate. Build the meal around that. Once you have your protein figured out, you can add vegetables, healthy fats, or carbs if there's room.

Protein Supplements: What Works and What Doesn't

Let's talk about protein powder because for a lot of people on GLP-1 medications, it becomes essential.

Not all protein powders are created equal. The main types are whey, casein, plant-based, and collagen. Each has pros and cons.

Whey protein is probably the most popular. It's derived from milk, it digests quickly, it tastes good in most cases, and it has a complete amino acid profile. It's great for post-workout or any time you need quick protein. The downside is that some people don't tolerate dairy well, especially when their digestion is already sensitive from GLP-1 medications. Whey isolate is a purer form with less lactose, so it might be easier on your stomach than whey concentrate.

Casein protein is also derived from milk, but it digests more slowly than whey. Some people like it before bed because it provides a steady release of amino acids overnight. It's thicker and creamier than whey, which can be good or bad depending on your preferences.

Plant-based protein powders are made from peas, rice, hemp, or a blend of plant sources. They're good for people who don't eat dairy or prefer plant-based options. The taste and texture can be hit or miss. Some brands are great, others are chalky and unpleasant. Plant proteins often need to be blended from multiple sources to get a complete amino acid profile, so look for blends rather than single-source options.

Collagen protein has become popular, but it's not ideal as your main protein source. Collagen is missing some essential amino acids, so it's not complete. It's fine as a supplement for skin, joints, and hair, but don't count it toward your daily protein goal for muscle preservation. Use whey, casein, or plant-based protein for that.

When choosing a protein powder, look for one with at least 20 grams of protein per serving, minimal added sugars, and ingredients you recognize. Some powders are loaded with artificial sweeteners, thickeners, and other additives that can upset your stomach, especially when you're on a GLP-1 medication.

Taste matters too. If it tastes terrible, you won't drink it. Try a few brands and flavors until you find one you can tolerate. Chocolate and vanilla are usually safe bets, but there are all kinds of flavors available now.

Ready-to-drink protein shakes are another option if you don't want to deal with mixing powder. Brands like Premier Protein, Fairlife Core Power, and Muscle Milk have shakes with 30 grams of protein that you can just grab and drink. They're more expensive than powder, but they're convenient.

Protein bars can work in a pinch, but they're usually not as protein-dense as shakes and they often contain more sugar and fat. They're fine occasionally, but they're not ideal as your primary protein source.

Before adding protein supplements to your routine, talk with your doctor, especially if you have any kidney issues, digestive conditions, or other health concerns that might be affected by increased protein intake.

Case Study: The Difference Adequate Protein Makes

Let me tell you about two clients who started GLP-1 medications at almost the same time. Both were women in their early 40s, both weighed around 190 pounds, both wanted to lose about 40 pounds. Their experiences were really different, and protein was a big part of why.

Client A didn't pay much attention to protein. She knew she should eat some, but it wasn't a priority. Her appetite was so suppressed that she was mostly eating whatever she could tolerate, which often meant carb-heavy foods like crackers, toast, fruit, and the occasional piece of chicken or cheese. She was probably averaging 40 to 50 grams of protein per day. She wasn't exercising much either.

Over six months, she lost 38 pounds. Amazing progress. But when we did a body composition scan, 16 of those pounds were muscle. She'd lost 22 pounds of fat and 16 pounds of muscle. She was frustrated because even at her goal weight, she didn't look the way she expected. She still felt soft and undefined. Her energy was lower than she thought it would be. And her weight loss had completely stalled in month five, which we realized was because her metabolism had dropped significantly from the muscle loss.

Client B took a different approach. From the start, we focused on protein. She aimed for 100 to 120 grams per day, which was challenging given her suppressed appetite. She had a protein shake every morning, prioritized chicken or fish at lunch and dinner, and snacked on Greek yogurt or hard-boiled eggs. She also did resistance training twice a week, which we'll talk more about in the next chapter.

Over the same six months, she also lost 38 pounds. But her body composition was very different. She lost 32 pounds of fat and only 6 pounds of muscle. She looked leaner and more toned at her goal weight. She felt strong. Her metabolism hadn't dropped nearly as much. And she was able to continue losing weight when she wanted to because her muscle mass was intact.

Same starting point, same ending weight, completely different outcomes. The main difference was protein intake and some resistance training.

I'm not saying protein is magic. But I am saying it's one of the most important factors in determining whether your weight loss leaves you better off or worse off in the long run.

Here's what I tell every client who starts a GLP-1

medication. If you can only focus on one thing besides taking your medication, make it protein. Not tracking every calorie, not eliminating certain foods, not doing hours of cardio. Just protein. Get enough protein every day, and you'll protect your muscle, your metabolism, and your long-term results.

It's not always easy when your appetite is gone. But it's worth the effort. Your future self will thank you.

In the next chapter, we'll talk about movement and exercise, which work hand-in-hand with protein to preserve muscle and maximize fat loss. But even if you don't exercise at all, adequate protein intake will still make a significant difference in your results.

Chapter 5
The Exercise Factor

Here's something I see all the time. Someone starts a GLP-1 medication, their appetite drops, the weight starts coming off, and they think, "Great, I don't need to exercise anymore. The medication is doing the work."

And honestly, I get it. When you've struggled with your weight for years and suddenly you have a tool that's actually working, it's tempting to let the medication carry all the weight. Plus, a lot of people feel more tired on these medications, at least initially. The idea of adding exercise on top of everything else feels like too much.

But here's the reality. The people who get the best results on GLP-1 medications, both in terms of how they look and how they feel, are the ones who keep moving. Exercise doesn't just help you lose weight faster. It changes what kind of weight you lose, how you feel during the process, and how sustainable your results are long-term.

Why GLP-1s Don't Eliminate the Need for Movement

The medication suppresses your appetite and helps you eat less. That's its job, and it does it well. But it doesn't build muscle. It doesn't strengthen your bones. It doesn't improve your cardiovascular health. It doesn't boost your mood or energy levels. Movement does all of those things.

When you lose weight without exercising, especially when you're losing it quickly, your body doesn't just burn fat. It also breaks down muscle tissue. We talked about this in the last chapter. Adequate protein helps protect muscle, but exercise takes that protection to another level. Exercise, particularly resistance training, sends a strong signal to your body that muscle is being used and needs to be maintained. Without that signal, your body has no reason to hold onto muscle when it's in an energy deficit.

There's also the metabolic piece. Exercise burns calories during the activity itself, sure. But it also increases your metabolic rate for hours afterward, especially if you're doing resistance training or higher-intensity cardio. And building or maintaining muscle through exercise keeps your resting metabolic rate higher long-term. All of that makes weight loss easier and weight maintenance more sustainable.

Beyond the physical benefits, movement affects how you feel. A lot of people on GLP-1 medications report feeling tired or low-energy, especially in the first few months. Exercise actually helps with that. It seems counterintuitive, but moving your body regularly tends to increase your energy levels over time. It also improves mood, reduces stress, and helps you sleep better.

And here's something people don't think about enough. If you lose a lot of weight without exercising, you're going to be smaller, but you're also going to be weaker. Your body composition won't be as good as it could be. You might hit your goal weight and still feel disappointed with how you look or how you feel physically. Exercise changes that equation.

Resistance Training: The Plateau-Breaker

If you can only do one type of exercise while you're on a GLP-1 medication, make it resistance training. Lifting weights, using resistance bands, doing bodyweight exercises. This is the most important type of movement for preserving muscle and improving body composition during weight loss.

Resistance training tells your body that your muscles are needed. When you lift weights or do other forms of resistance exercise, you create small amounts of damage to muscle fibers. Your body repairs that damage by rebuilding the muscle, assuming you're giving it adequate protein. This process protects existing muscle and, in some cases, can even build new muscle despite being in a calorie deficit.

Without resistance training, your body has no particular reason to keep muscle around when you're losing weight. Muscle is metabolically expensive. It requires energy to maintain. If you're not using it in a demanding way, your body will happily let it go to conserve energy.

I've seen this play out over and over. Two people lose the same amount of weight on the same medication. One does resistance training two or three times per week. The other doesn't exercise at all. The person who lifts weights looks leaner, more toned, and more defined at the same weight. They're also stronger, they have better posture, and their metabolism hasn't dropped as much.

Resistance training is also one of the best tools for breaking through plateaus. When weight loss stalls, adding or increasing resistance training can often get things moving again. It increases your metabolic rate, it builds metabolically active tissue, and it creates a strong stimulus for your body to prioritize fat loss over muscle loss.

You don't need to spend hours in the gym. Two to three sessions per week of 30 to 45 minutes each is enough for most people. Focus on compound movements that work multiple muscle groups at once. Squats, lunges, push-ups, rows, overhead presses, deadlifts. These exercises give you the most benefit for your time.

If you're new to resistance training, start with bodyweight exercises or light dumbbells. You don't need to lift heavy right away. Just get started with something manageable. As you get stronger, you can progressively increase the challenge. The key is consistency, not intensity.

If you have access to a gym, great. Use the machines, the free weights, whatever feels comfortable. If you don't have access to a gym, no problem. Bodyweight exercises and a set of resistance bands can be incredibly effective. There are countless YouTube videos and apps that can guide you through at-home workouts.

The important thing is to actually do it. Resistance training is the single most effective exercise tool for getting the body composition results you want on a GLP-1 medication.

Cardio: How Much Is Enough (And How Much Is Too Much)?

Cardio has its place, but it's not as critical as resistance training for people on GLP-1 medications. That might sound surprising since cardio is what most people think of when they think of exercise for weight loss.

Cardio does burn calories, which can help create or deepen your calorie deficit. It's good for cardiovascular health. It can improve your endurance and stamina. But it doesn't protect muscle the way resistance training does. And if you do too much cardio, especially without adequate protein and resistance training, you can actually accelerate muscle loss.

A reasonable approach for most people is to do moderate cardio two to four times per week for 20 to 40 minutes per session. This could be walking, cycling, swimming, using an elliptical, hiking, dancing, whatever you enjoy. The goal is to get your heart rate up and keep it elevated for a sustained period.

You don't need to do intense cardio unless you enjoy it. Long, grueling cardio sessions aren't necessary for weight loss on GLP-1 medications. In fact, doing too much intense cardio can backfire. It can increase hunger, which works against the appetite suppression from your medication. It can increase fatigue, which might make you less active overall. And it can promote muscle loss if you're not careful with protein and recovery.

If you like cardio and it makes you feel good, by all means, do it. But don't feel like you need to spend an hour on the treadmill every day. That's not the best use of your time or energy when you're trying to lose weight and preserve muscle.

One type of cardio that can be particularly effective is high-intensity interval training, or HIIT. This involves short bursts of intense effort followed by recovery periods. For example, sprinting for 30 seconds, then walking for 90 seconds, and repeating that cycle for 15 to 20 minutes. HIIT burns a lot of calories in a short time, and it has been shown to preserve muscle better than steady-state cardio. But it's also more demanding, so it's not appropriate for everyone, especially if you're just starting out or dealing with low energy from the medication.

The bottom line on cardio is this. Some is good. More isn't necessarily better. Prioritize resistance training first, then add cardio as your energy and schedule allow.

NEAT (Non-Exercise Activity Thermogenesis): The Hidden Calorie Burner

Here's something most people don't think about. The calories you burn during formal exercise, whether that's lifting weights or doing cardio, make up a relatively small portion of your total daily energy expenditure. For most people, exercise accounts for maybe 10 to 20% of total calories burned, and that's if you're exercising regularly.

The biggest chunk of your daily calorie burn is your basal metabolic rate, the energy your body uses just to keep you alive. But there's another significant category that often gets overlooked. It's called NEAT, which stands for Non-Exercise Activity Thermogenesis. This is all the movement you do throughout the day that isn't formal exercise. Walking to your car, taking the stairs, doing housework, fidgeting, standing while you work, carrying groceries, playing with your kids or pets. All of that adds up.

For some people, NEAT can account for several hundred calories per day. The difference between someone with high NEAT and someone with low NEAT can be 300 to 500 calories per day or more. That's huge. Over a week, that's the equivalent of burning an extra pound of fat.

Here's why this matters for people on GLP-1 medications. A lot of people become less active overall when they start these drugs. They feel more tired. They have less energy. And because the weight is coming off anyway, they don't feel motivated to move as much. They start sitting more, moving less, taking the elevator instead of the stairs. Their NEAT drops significantly.

This is a problem for a few reasons. Lower NEAT means fewer calories burned, which can slow weight loss or contribute to plateaus. It also means less muscle activation throughout the day, which doesn't help with muscle preservation. And it can contribute to feeling even more tired and sluggish, creating a negative cycle.

The good news is that increasing NEAT doesn't require structured exercise. It just requires being more active in your daily life.

Park farther away from store entrances. Take the stairs instead of the elevator when it's an option. Stand while you're on the phone or watching TV. Walk around while you're waiting for something. Set a timer to get up and move every hour if you have a desk job. Do a lap around your house or office between tasks. Dance while you're cooking. Play more actively with your kids or pets. Find reasons to move instead of reasons to sit.

These little movements might seem insignificant, but they add up to hundreds of extra calories burned over the course of a day. And unlike formal exercise, they don't require motivation or willpower or getting dressed to go to the gym. They're just part of how you live your life.

One simple strategy is to track your daily steps. Most smartphones do this automatically. Aim for at least 7,000 to 10,000 steps per day. If you're currently averaging 3,000 steps, don't jump straight to 10,000. Add 1,000 steps per week until you reach your goal. It's an easy way to ensure you're maintaining a baseline level of activity.

NEAT won't replace the benefits of resistance training or cardio. But it's a powerful tool for increasing your total daily energy expenditure without much extra effort.

Exercise Timing and Appetite Suppression

Here's something interesting about exercise and GLP-1 medications. Exercise can temporarily affect your appetite, but the medication tends to override those effects.

Normally, intense exercise might suppress appetite for a short period afterward, while lighter exercise might stimulate appetite. But when you're on a GLP-1 medication, your appetite is already so suppressed that exercise doesn't change it much. Most people find they're not any hungrier after working out than they were before.

This can actually be an advantage. You don't have to worry as much about exercise making you ravenously hungry and undoing your calorie deficit. The medication keeps your appetite in check regardless of your activity level.

The challenge is making sure you're eating enough to fuel your workouts and recover properly, especially if you're doing resistance training. If you're not hungry but you've just done a demanding workout, you still need to eat. Your body needs protein to repair muscle tissue and carbohydrates to replenish energy stores. Don't skip meals just because you're not hungry. Stick to your eating schedule and prioritize protein, even on days when you exercise.

Some people find that exercising in the morning works well because it can boost energy for the rest of the day. Others prefer evening workouts as a way to wind down. There's no perfect time to exercise. The best time is whenever you're most likely to actually do it consistently.

One consideration is the timing of your GLP-1 injection relative to exercise. Some people feel more nauseated or fatigued in the day or two after their injection. If that's you, you might want to schedule lighter workouts during that window and save more intense sessions for when you're feeling better. It's all about listening to your body and adjusting as needed.

Building Sustainable Movement Habits

The key to making exercise work long-term isn't finding the perfect workout program. It's finding something you can actually stick with.

A lot of people approach exercise with an all-or-nothing mindset. They decide they're going to work out six days a week for an hour each time. They do it for two weeks, burn out, and quit. Then they feel guilty and don't exercise at all for months. That pattern doesn't help anyone.

Start with something manageable. If you're not currently exercising at all, don't commit to five days a week right out of the gate. Start with two days a week. Make it something simple and achievable. Two 30-minute resistance training sessions. That's it. Do that consistently for a month. Once it feels like a normal part of your routine, you can add more if you want.

Choose activities you don't hate. You don't have to love exercise, but if you absolutely despise what you're doing, you won't keep doing it. If you hate running, don't run. If you hate gyms, work out at home. If you find lifting weights boring, try a fitness class or a sport. There are so many options for movement. Find something that feels tolerable, maybe even enjoyable.

Make it convenient. The easier it is to exercise, the more likely you are to do it. If you have to drive 30 minutes to a gym, that's a barrier. If you can work out at home in 20 minutes, that's easier to fit into your life. Remove as many obstacles as possible.

Schedule it like an appointment. Don't just plan to exercise "when you have time." You'll never have time. Put it on your calendar. Treat it like you would a doctor's appointment or a work meeting. It's not optional. It's part of your routine.

Track your progress in some way. Maybe you keep a simple log of your workouts. Maybe you note how much weight you're lifting or how many steps you're taking. Maybe you take progress photos or measurements. Seeing tangible evidence that you're getting stronger or more capable is motivating and helps you stay consistent.

Be flexible and forgiving with yourself. Life happens. You'll miss workouts sometimes. That's okay. Don't let one missed session turn into a month of inactivity. Just get back to it as soon as you can. Consistency over time matters more than perfection in any given week.

The Danger of Becoming Sedentary on GLP-1s

Let me paint a picture of what can happen if you become too sedentary while losing weight on these medications.

You start the medication. Your appetite drops. You're eating less. The weight starts coming off, which is great. But you're also feeling tired, so you're moving less. You're sitting more, walking less, definitely not exercising. Your daily activity drops significantly.

Because you're not doing any resistance training and you're not eating much protein, a large portion of your weight loss is muscle. Over several months, you lose 40 pounds. But 15 of those pounds are muscle. Your metabolism has slowed considerably, both from the weight loss and from the muscle loss.

You're smaller, sure. But you're also weaker. You get winded going up stairs. Your posture is poor because your core and back muscles have atrophied. You feel tired all the time. Your body composition isn't what you hoped for. You still have more body fat than you expected at this weight because you lost so much muscle along with the fat.

Now let's say you stop the medication at some point, either because you've reached your goal or because you can't afford it anymore or because of side effects. Your appetite comes back. But your metabolism is much slower than it was before you started because of all the muscle you lost. You start regaining weight quickly. Within a year, you've gained back most or all of what you lost, and you're in a worse metabolic position than when you started.

This is not an exaggeration. I've seen this happen. It's heartbreaking, and it's preventable.

The alternative is staying active throughout the weight loss process. You do some resistance training. You keep your daily activity up. You prioritize protein. You lose the same 40 pounds, but you only lose 5 pounds of muscle. You feel strong. You have energy. Your body composition is great. Your metabolism is in a much better place.

If you stop the medication, your appetite returns, but you're in a better position to maintain your weight because your metabolism hasn't tanked. You've built habits around movement and nutrition that help you sustain your results. Even if you gain back a few pounds, you're still way ahead of where you started.

Movement isn't optional if you want the best outcomes from GLP-1 medications. It's essential. Not because the medication doesn't work without it. It does. But because the quality of your results and your ability to maintain those results long-term depends on staying active.

You don't have to become a gym rat or a marathon runner. You just need to move your body regularly in ways that challenge your muscles and keep you active throughout the day. That's enough to make a massive difference.

In the next section of this book, we'll get into more advanced troubleshooting strategies. But before we move on, make sure you've got these fundamentals covered. Energy balance, protein, and movement. Those three things form the foundation. If any of them are missing or inconsistent, the advanced strategies won't help nearly as much. Get these basics right, and you'll be amazed at how much better your results become.

PART 3

Advanced Troubleshooting Strategies

Chapter 6
When You're a Slow Responder (First 3 Months)

A client sent me a frustrated text message six weeks after starting tirzepatide. "I've only lost four pounds. Everyone else I know has lost at least ten by now. Should I just quit?"

I understood her frustration. When you start a medication that's supposed to help with weight loss, and you hear stories about people dropping twenty pounds in two months, losing four pounds feels like failure. But here's what I told her, and what I want you to know if you're in a similar situation. Slow doesn't mean it's not working. And there are usually specific, fixable reasons why your response is slower than you'd like.

Let's figure out what those reasons might be.

Defining "Slow Response": What's Normal vs. Concerning

First, we need to establish what a typical response actually looks like so you can tell if you're genuinely a slow responder or if your expectations just don't match reality.

In clinical trials, people taking semaglutide lost an average of about 5 to 6% of their body weight in the first three months. For someone weighing 200 pounds, that's 10 to 12 pounds. People taking tirzepatide lost slightly more, around 6 to 8% in the first three months, which would be 12 to 16 pounds for that same person.

Those are averages. Some people lose more, some lose less. If you're losing around 5 to 7% of your body weight in the first three months, you're having a pretty typical response. That might feel slow compared to the dramatic stories you hear, but it's actually right in line with what the research shows.

A slow response would be losing less than 5% of your body weight after three months on a therapeutic dose. For that 200-pound person, that would be less than 10 pounds. If you're in that range, it's worth investigating why.

A concerning response would be losing less than 2 to 3% of your body weight after three months, or essentially no weight loss at all despite being on an adequate dose. That suggests either the medication isn't working for you, or there are significant factors interfering with your response.

Keep in mind that weight loss isn't linear. You might lose three pounds one week, nothing the next week, then two pounds the following week. What matters is the overall trend over weeks and months, not day-to-day or even week-to-week fluctuations.

Also, remember that these medications are typically started at low doses and gradually increased over several weeks or months. You might not be on a full therapeutic dose yet in the first month or two. If you're still in the titration phase, slower weight loss is completely normal and expected.

Patience vs. Problem-Solving: When to Give It Time

This is the tricky balance. You don't want to be impatient and make changes too quickly. But you also don't want to waste months being too passive if there's actually a problem.

Here's a reasonable framework. If you're in the first four to six weeks and you're still titrating up to a therapeutic dose, give it time. Your dose is probably too low to produce dramatic results yet. Be patient. Focus on building good habits around protein and movement. Don't panic about the scale.

If you're eight to twelve weeks in and you're on what should be a therapeutic dose but you've lost less than 5% of your body weight, it's time to start troubleshooting. Not panicking, but actively looking for reasons why your response might be slower than expected.

If you're three months in on a full dose and you've lost less than 2 to 3% of your body weight, you need to have a conversation with your doctor. Something is either wrong with how you're taking the medication, or there are significant underlying factors at play, or the medication simply isn't effective for you.

The key is giving yourself enough time to see what the medication can do, while also being proactive about addressing issues that might be holding you back. Patience doesn't mean doing nothing. It means being strategic about when and how you intervene.

Are You Actually on a Therapeutic Dose? Understanding Titration

This is one of the most common reasons people think they're slow responders when actually they're just not on a high enough dose yet.

GLP-1 medications are almost always started at a low dose and gradually increased over time. This titration process helps your body adjust to the medication and minimizes side effects. But it also means you might spend several weeks or even months on doses that aren't high enough to produce significant weight loss.

For semaglutide (Ozempic or Wegovy), the typical titration looks like this. You start at 0.25 mg per week for four weeks. Then you increase to 0.5 mg per week for four weeks. Then 1 mg per week for four weeks. Then 1.7 mg if you're on Wegovy. Finally, you might go up to 2.4 mg, which is the full dose for weight loss.

That means it could take three to four months just to reach the full therapeutic dose. If you're only two months in and you're on 0.5 or 1 mg, you haven't even gotten to the dose where most people see their best results. Your "slow response" might just be that you're not on a high enough dose yet.

For tirzepatide (Mounjaro or Zepbound), the titration is similar. You start at 2.5 mg per week for four weeks, then increase to 5 mg for four weeks, then 7.5 mg, then 10 mg, and potentially up to 12.5 or 15 mg. Again, it takes months to reach higher doses.

If you're frustrated with your progress, check what dose you're on and how long you've been at that dose. If you just increased two weeks ago, give it more time. The full effect of a dose increase often takes three to four weeks to show up.

If you've been on the same dose for two months and you're not seeing results, that's when you should talk to your doctor about whether it's time to increase. But don't make that decision on your own. Dose changes need to be guided by your healthcare provider.

Injection Technique: Are You Doing It Correctly? Does Switching Injection Sites Help?

Believe it or not, how you inject the medication can affect how well it works. If you're not injecting correctly, you might not be absorbing the medication properly.

GLP-1 medications are injected subcutaneously, which means into the fat layer just under your skin, not into muscle. The most common injection sites are your abdomen, thighs, and the back of your upper arms. Some people also use their buttocks.

Here's what correct technique looks like. Clean the injection site with an alcohol wipe and let it dry. Pinch a fold of skin to create a small mound. Insert the needle at a 90-degree angle into the pinched skin. Press the button to inject and hold it for about five to ten seconds to make sure all the medication is delivered. Then remove the needle and release the pinched skin.

Common mistakes include not holding the button long enough, injecting too quickly, injecting at the wrong angle, or injecting into the same exact spot repeatedly.

Rotating injection sites is important. If you inject into the same spot over and over, you can develop areas of thickened or hardened tissue. This can affect how well the medication is absorbed. Try to rotate through different areas. If you inject in your abdomen one week, use your thigh the next week, then your other thigh, then back to your abdomen. Within each area, vary the specific spot you're using.

Some people find they respond better to certain injection sites. The abdomen tends to have the most consistent absorption for most people. Thighs can be a bit slower to absorb. Arms are trickier to self-inject but work fine for some people. If you've been injecting in one area consistently and not seeing great results, try switching to a different site for a few weeks to see if it makes a difference.

Temperature can also affect absorption. If you inject into

cold skin, absorption might be slower. Make sure the injection site is at normal body temperature before you inject. If you've been outside in cold weather or your skin feels cool, wait a bit or warm up the area before injecting.

If you're using a pre-filled pen, make sure you're priming it correctly before your first injection. Most pens need to be primed to remove air bubbles. Check the instructions that came with your medication to make sure you're doing this step.

Medication Storage and Handling Issues

This is something people often overlook. If your medication isn't stored properly, it might not work as well as it should.

GLP-1 medications need to be refrigerated before first use. They should be stored at 36 to 46 degrees Fahrenheit, which is standard refrigerator temperature. Don't freeze them. Freezing can damage the medication and make it ineffective. If your medication accidentally freezes, don't use it. Get a replacement.

Once you start using a pen, most GLP-1 medications can be stored at room temperature or in the refrigerator for a certain period, usually 28 to 56 days depending on the specific medication. Check your medication's instructions for the exact timeframe. After that time, even if there's medication left in the pen, you need to discard it and start a new one.

Don't leave your medication in a hot car, in direct sunlight, or anywhere it might get too warm. Heat can degrade the medication. If you're traveling, use a cooling case or keep it in a refrigerator whenever possible.

Check the medication before you inject. It should be clear and colorless or slightly yellow depending on the specific drug. If it looks cloudy, discolored, or has particles floating in it, don't use it. That could mean it's been contaminated or has degraded.

If you're using compounded semaglutide or tirzepatide from a compounding pharmacy, storage requirements might be different. Follow the instructions provided by the pharmacy. Compounded medications sometimes have shorter shelf lives or different storage needs than brand-name versions.

If you've been storing your medication improperly, that could absolutely affect how well it's working. Get a new pen, make sure you store it correctly, and see if your response improves.

Food Timing Around Injections

Some people wonder if eating around the time of their injection affects how well the medication works. The short answer is no, not really. But there are some considerations.

For injected GLP-1 medications like semaglutide and tirzepatide, it doesn't matter if you inject on an empty stomach or after eating. The medication is absorbed from the injection site, not from your digestive system. Food in your stomach doesn't interfere with that absorption.

That said, some people feel more nauseated if they inject shortly after eating a large meal. If nausea is an issue for you, you might want to inject when your stomach is relatively empty or at least not overly full. But this is about comfort, not effectiveness.

There's also the oral version of semaglutide, Rybelsus, which is a different story. That one does need to be taken on an empty stomach, and you need to wait 30 minutes before eating or drinking anything other than water. If you're on Rybelsus and you're not following those instructions, that could definitely affect your results.

For injectable versions, the main thing is consistency. Pick a day and time that works for you and stick with it as much as possible. Some people like to inject on the same day each week at the same time. Others are more flexible. Either approach is fine as long as you're taking your dose weekly.

If you miss a dose, the general guidance is to take it as soon as you remember, as long as your next dose isn't within two days. If your next dose is in less than two days, skip the missed dose and just take your next one on schedule. Don't double up. Check with your doctor if you're unsure what to do about a missed dose.

Hydration and Its Surprising Impact
This is something that doesn't get talked about enough.

Hydration can actually affect how you respond to GLP-1 medications, both in terms of weight loss and side effects.

When you're eating less food, you're also getting less water from food. A lot of hydration comes from what we eat, not just what we drink. Fruits, vegetables, soups, even cooked grains contain significant amounts of water. If your food intake has dropped dramatically, your water intake from food has dropped too.

GLP-1 medications can also slow digestion, which can affect how your body processes fluids. And some of the common side effects, like nausea or diarrhea, can lead to dehydration if you're not careful.

Dehydration can make you feel more tired, which might make you less active, which can slow weight loss. It can make side effects like nausea and constipation worse. It can even affect how well your body mobilizes and burns fat. Adequate hydration is important for metabolic processes.

A good rule of thumb is to drink at least eight glasses of water per day, and more if you're active or it's hot outside. Your urine should be pale yellow. If it's dark yellow, you need more water.

Some people find that drinking water before meals helps them feel fuller faster, which can be helpful. Others find that drinking too much during meals makes them feel uncomfortably full when they're already dealing with appetite suppression. Experiment and see what works for you.

If you're struggling with nausea, sipping water throughout the day can help. So can drinking ginger tea or adding a little lemon to your water. Just make sure you're getting enough fluids.

Dehydration can also cause the scale to show false plateaus. If you're dehydrated, you might be losing fat but retaining less water, which masks fat loss on the scale. Then when you rehydrate, the scale jumps up even though you haven't gained fat. Staying consistently hydrated helps you get more accurate readings on the scale.

Sleep, Stress, and Cortisol's Role

Here's where we get into factors that a lot of people don't connect to weight loss, but they matter more than you might think.

Poor sleep can significantly slow weight loss. When you don't sleep enough, your body produces more ghrelin, which is a hunger hormone, and less leptin, which is a satiety hormone. GLP-1 medications help counteract this to some degree, but they don't completely override the effects of sleep deprivation.

Lack of sleep also increases cortisol, which is a stress hormone. Elevated cortisol can promote fat storage, particularly around your midsection. It can increase insulin resistance, which makes fat loss harder. It can also increase cravings for high-calorie comfort foods, which you might give in to even if your appetite is generally suppressed.

Aim for seven to nine hours of quality sleep per night. If you're consistently getting less than that, it could be slowing your progress. Work on improving your sleep hygiene. Keep your bedroom cool and dark. Avoid screens for an hour before bed. Establish a consistent sleep schedule. If you have a sleep disorder like sleep apnea, get it treated. Quality sleep is not optional for optimal weight loss.

Chronic stress is another huge factor. When you're stressed, your body produces more cortisol. We just talked about what cortisol does. High cortisol levels over extended periods can make weight loss extremely difficult, even with medication.

Stress also tends to increase emotional eating. Even with appetite suppression, you might find yourself reaching for food when you're stressed, anxious, or overwhelmed. The medication reduces physical hunger, but it doesn't eliminate emotional eating triggers.

Finding ways to manage stress is important. Exercise helps. So does prayer, meditation, deep breathing, spending time in nature, connecting with friends, engaging in hobbies you enjoy. Therapy can be helpful if stress is a major issue in your life. Don't underestimate the impact that chronic stress can have on your ability to lose weight.

Questions to Ask Your Doctor (Without Asking to Increase Dose Prematurely)

If you're concerned about your response to the medication, there are productive ways to have that conversation with your doctor. You don't want to come across as demanding or impatient, but you also want to make sure any potential issues are addressed.

Here are some good questions to ask:

"I've been on this dose for X weeks. Is this long enough to evaluate whether it's working for me, or should I give it more time?"

This shows that you understand titration takes time, but you're checking in about whether you've given the current dose a fair shot.

"I've lost X pounds so far. Is that in the range of what you'd expect at this point, or is it lower than typical?"

This helps you understand if your response is genuinely slow or if your expectations are just off.

"Are there any lab tests we should run to see if there's an underlying issue affecting my response? Things like thyroid function, insulin levels, or cortisol?"

This shows you're thinking systematically about potential barriers to weight loss, not just asking for a higher dose.

"I want to make sure I'm taking the medication correctly. Can we review my injection technique?"

This demonstrates that you're taking responsibility for your part in the process.

"Are there any medications I'm taking that might interfere with the GLP-1? Or any medical conditions that might affect how I respond?"

This is a smart question that many doctors will appreciate.

"What should I be focusing on in terms of diet and exercise to get the best results from this medication?"

This shows you understand that the medication is just one tool and you're willing to do the work on the lifestyle side.

"If I'm still not seeing the results we'd hope for after another month, what would be the next step? Would we increase the dose, or consider other options?"

This frames the conversation about next steps without demanding immediate action.

Approach the conversation as a partnership. Your doctor wants you to succeed. But they also need to make sure you're on the medication long enough at each dose, that you're handling the basics like protein and movement, and that there aren't other factors at play before jumping to increase your dose.

Being a slow responder in the first few months doesn't mean the medication won't work for you. It might mean you need a higher dose eventually. It might mean you need to tighten up the fundamentals around nutrition and exercise. It might mean there are other factors that need to be addressed. But it rarely means you should give up.

Stay patient, stay proactive, and work with your doctor to figure out what adjustments might help. Most people who start as slow responders can improve their results with the right troubleshooting.

Chapter 7
The Plateau: When Weight Loss Stops

Three months ago, a client was on top of the world. She'd lost twenty-eight pounds on semaglutide and was feeling incredible. Then the scale just stopped moving. For five weeks, nothing. Same dose, same habits, same everything. But zero weight loss.

She was convinced something had gone wrong. Maybe the medication stopped working. Maybe her body had adapted. Maybe she'd never lose another pound. She was ready to give up.

Here's what I told her, and what I need you to understand if you're in the same situation. Plateaus are not failures. They're a normal, predictable part of weight loss. And more importantly, they're usually temporary and fixable.

Why Plateaus Happen (They're Actually Normal)

Let's start with the basic truth. Almost everyone who loses

a significant amount of weight will hit at least one plateau, and often several. It doesn't matter if you're on medication or not. It doesn't matter how perfectly you're doing everything. Plateaus happen because your body is constantly adapting to your new weight and your reduced calorie intake.

When you start losing weight, especially in the first few weeks or months, progress tends to be fairly steady. Your body hasn't fully adjusted yet. The calorie deficit you've created is significant. The weight comes off at a predictable pace.

But as time goes on, things change. You weigh less now, which means your body requires fewer calories to maintain itself. Remember, a smaller body needs less energy than a larger body. So the calorie deficit that worked great when you weighed 200 pounds might not be much of a deficit anymore at 175 pounds.

Your body also becomes more efficient at using energy. This is metabolic adaptation, which we'll talk about in detail in the next section. Basically, your body learns to function on fewer calories. It becomes stingy with energy expenditure. This is a survival mechanism, and it's completely normal.

Your activity level might have decreased without you realizing it. You're eating less, so you have less energy. You might be moving less throughout the day. Your workouts might be less intense than they used to be. All of that adds up to fewer calories burned.

Plateaus can also happen because you've gotten a bit loose

with the fundamentals. Maybe you were tracking your food religiously at first, but now you're eyeballing portions and they've crept up. Maybe you were strict about protein initially, but now you're having more days where you don't hit your target. Small inconsistencies accumulate over time.

The point is, plateaus are a sign that your body has adapted to what you've been doing. They're not a sign that the medication stopped working or that you'll never lose weight again. They're just your body's way of saying that what worked before needs to be adjusted now.

Metabolic Adaptation: Your Body's Defense Mechanism

Let's dig into what metabolic adaptation actually is, because understanding it helps you deal with plateaus without panicking.

Your body doesn't understand that you're trying to lose weight on purpose. It doesn't know you're taking medication or following a plan. All it knows is that energy coming in has been less than energy going out for an extended period, and body mass has been dropping. From your body's perspective, that's a threat.

Throughout human history, losing weight rapidly usually meant starvation, illness, or famine. Those are dangerous situations. So your body has evolved powerful mechanisms to slow weight loss and conserve energy when it perceives this threat.

One mechanism is reducing your resting metabolic rate beyond what you'd expect from weight loss alone. Yes, weighing less means you burn fewer calories. But metabolic adaptation means you burn even fewer calories than you should for your new weight. Your body becomes more efficient. It reduces energy spent on things like maintaining body temperature, digestion, and cellular repair. It does this to stretch the available energy as far as possible.

Another mechanism is reducing spontaneous movement. You fidget less. You take fewer steps throughout the day without consciously deciding to move less. Your NEAT drops. Again, this is your body trying to conserve energy.

Hormones shift too. Leptin, which signals that you have adequate energy stores, decreases. Ghrelin, which stimulates hunger, increases. Thyroid hormones can decrease slightly, which slows metabolism. All of these changes work together to make continued weight loss harder.

This isn't your body betraying you. It's your body trying to protect you from what it perceives as a threat. The problem is that in our modern environment with abundant food, this adaptation works against your goals.

The good news is that metabolic adaptation is partially reversible. When you eat more again, your metabolism speeds back up to some degree. When you take breaks from dieting, hormone levels improve. Your body doesn't stay in that low-energy state forever if you give it a break.

GLP-1 medications help by continuing to suppress appetite even when these adaptive mechanisms are trying to increase hunger. But they don't prevent metabolic adaptation entirely. Your metabolism will still slow down to some extent. You just won't feel as hungry as you would without the medication.

The Difference Between a True Plateau and Normal Fluctuations

Before you decide you've hit a plateau, you need to make sure you're actually at a plateau and not just experiencing normal weight fluctuations.

Your body weight changes daily based on water retention, digestion, hormones, sodium intake, carbohydrate intake, stress, exercise, and about a dozen other factors. You can easily fluctuate three to five pounds in either direction over the course of a few days without gaining or losing any actual fat.

Women especially see fluctuations related to their menstrual cycle. Water retention increases in the days leading up to your period. The scale might go up two to four pounds even though you haven't gained fat. Then once your period starts, that water weight drops off and you might see a sudden whoosh of weight loss.

High-sodium meals can cause temporary water retention. A big restaurant meal with lots of salt might make the scale jump up the next day, but it's water, not fat. A hard workout can cause temporary water retention as your muscles hold onto fluid for repair. Eating more carbs than usual can cause water retention because carbs are stored with water in your muscles.

All of this is normal. It's not a plateau. It's just your body doing what bodies do.

A true plateau is when your weight doesn't change at all, or changes minimally, over a sustained period despite consistent habits. We're talking three to four weeks at a minimum. If the scale has been bouncing around the same two or three pound range for a month or more, that's a plateau. If the scale went up two pounds this week after going down a pound last week, that's just fluctuation.

The best way to identify a true plateau is to look at the trend over time, not day-to-day numbers. Weigh yourself at the same time under the same conditions, ideally first thing in the morning after using the bathroom and before eating. Track that weight over weeks. If the trend line has been flat for a month or more, you're probably at a plateau. If it's still trending downward even with ups and downs along the way, you're fine.

How Long Should You Wait Before Taking Action?

This is the million-dollar question. How long do you wait before deciding the plateau is real and you need to do something about it?

My general rule is four weeks. If your weight hasn't moved

at all, or has only moved by a pound or less, for four full weeks, and you've been consistent with your habits, then it's time to start troubleshooting.

Why four weeks? Because that's long enough to account for normal fluctuations, hormonal cycles, and temporary water retention. But it's not so long that you've wasted months spinning your wheels.

If you jump into action after one or two weeks of no movement, you're probably reacting to normal fluctuation, not a real plateau. You might make unnecessary changes that complicate things or create problems that didn't exist.

But if you wait too long, you can lose motivation and momentum. Sitting at the same weight for two or three months without doing anything is demoralizing. And the longer you plateau, the harder it can be to break through.

So four weeks is the sweet spot. Give it four weeks of consistency. If nothing changes, then it's time to try something different.

During those four weeks, make sure you're actually being consistent. Are you tracking your food accurately? Are you hitting your protein targets most days? Are you exercising regularly? Are you getting adequate sleep? Are you managing stress? If any of those things have slipped, tighten them up first before deciding you need a more dramatic intervention.

Often, what looks like a plateau is actually just inconsistency that's harder to see. Weekend eating that's gotten a bit loose.

A few extra snacks here and there that you're not accounting for. Workouts that have become less intense. Protein intake that's dropped. Fix those things first. See if that gets the scale moving again. If you tighten everything up for two to three weeks and still see no movement, then you're dealing with a true plateau that needs a different approach.

Dealing With the Emotional Side of Plateaus

Before we dive into strategies for breaking plateaus, let's talk about the emotional piece. Plateaus can be really demoralizing. You're doing everything right, but the scale won't budge. It's easy to feel discouraged, frustrated, or like giving up entirely.

First, remind yourself that plateaus don't mean failure. They're a normal part of the process. Almost everyone who loses significant weight experiences them. You're not doing anything wrong. Your body is just adapting.

Second, focus on non-scale victories during this time. Are your clothes fitting better? Do you have more energy? Are you sleeping better? Is your blood pressure improving? Are you feeling stronger? These things matter just as much as the number on the scale. Sometimes your body is changing in positive ways even when the scale isn't moving.

Third, remember that this is temporary. Plateaus eventually break if you stay consistent and make strategic adjustments. The worst thing you can do is give up during a plateau and undo all your progress. Stay the course.

It can help to take a mental break from the scale during a plateau. If weighing yourself daily is making you crazy, switch to weekly or even less frequent weigh-ins. Focus on the behaviors you can control rather than the outcome you can't control right now.

Talk to supportive people about what you're experiencing. Whether that's friends, family, a coach, or an online community. Knowing that others have been through the same thing and come out the other side can make a big difference.

And give yourself some grace. Weight loss is hard. Plateaus are frustrating. It's okay to feel disappointed. Just don't let that disappointment turn into a reason to quit.

Diet Breaks: The Counterintuitive Strategy

This is one of the most powerful tools for breaking plateaus, but it feels wrong to a lot of people. Taking a break from your deficit seems like it would slow progress, not help it. But the research and real-world experience both show that planned diet breaks can actually improve long-term weight loss.

Here's how it works. You've been in a calorie deficit for weeks or months. Your body has adapted. Your metabolism has slowed. Your hormones have shifted. Your energy is low. Everything is working against continued weight loss.

A diet break is a period of time, usually one to two weeks, where you eat at maintenance calories instead of a deficit. You're not eating in a surplus and you're not bingeing. You're eating enough to maintain your current weight, no more, no less.

This gives your body a break from the stress of being in a deficit. Your metabolism speeds up a bit. Leptin increases. Thyroid hormones improve. Energy levels recover. Psychologically, it also gives you a mental break from the restriction, which can help with long-term adherence.

After the diet break, you go back into your deficit. But now your body is in a better position to respond. The metabolic adaptation has been partially reversed. You might find that weight loss picks up again.

A proper diet break means calculating your maintenance calories for your current weight and activity level, then eating that amount consistently for one to two weeks. You're still tracking. You're still hitting protein targets. You're still exercising. You're just eating more than you were during your deficit phase.

This isn't a cheat week. You're not eating whatever you want. You're eating in a controlled, intentional way to give your body a break while minimizing fat regain.

For most people, a diet break every eight to twelve weeks makes sense if you're doing an extended period of weight loss. It helps prevent severe metabolic adaptation and keeps you mentally fresh.

On GLP-1 medications, diet breaks can be challenging because your appetite is so suppressed that eating at maintenance might feel uncomfortable. You might need to intentionally include more calorie-dense foods to reach your target without feeling overly full. But it's worth the effort if you've been plateaued for a while.

Refeed Days vs. Cheat Days

These terms get used interchangeably sometimes, but they're actually different concepts. Understanding the difference matters.

A refeed day is a planned, strategic day where you eat more than usual, particularly more carbohydrates, to give your body a temporary break from the deficit and boost leptin levels. It's controlled. You might increase your calories by 300 to 500 for the day, mostly from carbs. You're still hitting protein targets. You're still making reasonable food choices. It's intentional and structured.

Refeed days can help with metabolic adaptation and can improve workout performance. Some people do one refeed day per week, others do them less frequently. The idea is that the temporary increase in calories and carbs sends a signal to your body that food is available and it doesn't need to conserve energy so aggressively.

A cheat day, on the other hand, is usually unstructured. You eat whatever you want, however much you want. There's no tracking. There's no limit. It's a free-for-all. For some people, cheat days are psychologically helpful because they provide relief from the feeling of restriction. But they can also backfire.

On a true cheat day where you go all out, you can easily consume 3,000 to 5,000 calories or more. If you're in a 500-calorie daily deficit the rest of the week, that's a 3,500-calorie weekly deficit. One big cheat day can wipe out most or all of your weekly deficit, leaving you with minimal weight loss or even a slight gain for the week.

Cheat days also tend to trigger cravings and make it harder to get back on track the next day. You might find yourself wanting more of those foods for days afterward. It can set up a cycle of restriction and bingeing that's not healthy.

On GLP-1 medications, cheat days are usually less of an issue because your appetite is suppressed. You physically can't eat as much as you could before, even on a day when you're trying to indulge. But you can still eat enough to significantly slow your progress.

My recommendation is to skip the cheat day concept entirely. If you want to use strategic refeeds, do it in a controlled way. If you want to include foods you enjoy, work them into your regular eating in reasonable portions rather than saving them all up for one explosive day.

Reverse Dieting on GLP-1s

Reverse dieting is a strategy where you gradually increase calorie intake after extended dieting to help your metabolism recover. The typical approach is adding 100 to 200 calories per week until you reach maintenance levels.

On GLP-1 medications, this strategy can be useful if you've been plateaued for a while and your calories have gotten very low. Let's say you've been eating 1,200 calories per day for months and feel terrible. Gradually increasing to 1,500 or 1,600 calories over several weeks might help your metabolism recover enough that weight loss actually resumes at the higher intake.

It seems counterintuitive, but it works for some people. The key is monitoring your weight and how you feel during the process. If weight stays stable or drops slightly as you add calories back, you're on the right track.

This strategy works best with guidance from someone who understands the process well, like a dietitian or coach who specializes in metabolic recovery.

In the next chapter, we'll talk about nutritional optimization beyond just calories and protein. There are other dietary factors that can affect your progress, especially if you're dealing with a stubborn plateau or slow response.

Chapter 8
Nutritional Optimization

A client came to me frustrated after four months on Wegovy. She'd lost eighteen pounds, which was progress, but she felt terrible. She was constantly tired, her hair was thinning, her nails were brittle, and she was dealing with digestive issues she'd never had before. When we looked at what she was eating, the problem became clear. She was hitting around 1,200 calories per day, but those calories were coming from a very narrow range of foods. Mostly chicken, rice, and protein shakes. She was missing huge chunks of essential nutrients.

Once we diversified her diet and added some strategic supplements, everything changed. Her energy came back. Her hair stopped falling out. Her digestion improved. And interestingly, her weight loss actually picked up again.

This chapter is about going beyond just calories and protein. Those are the foundation, but they're not the whole picture. The quality and variety of what you eat matters, especially when you're eating less overall.

Micronutrients: What You Might Be Missing

When you're eating significantly less food than you used to, you're also getting significantly fewer vitamins and minerals. This is one of the hidden challenges of rapid weight loss on GLP-1 medications.

Your body needs dozens of different micronutrients to function properly. Vitamins, minerals, antioxidants. They're involved in everything from energy production to immune function to hormone regulation to bone health. When you're eating 2,500 calories a day, it's relatively easy to get enough of these nutrients just by eating a varied diet. When you're eating 1,200 to 1,500 calories a day and you can barely stomach certain foods, getting adequate micronutrients becomes much harder.

Some of the most common deficiencies I see in people on GLP-1 medications include iron, vitamin D, vitamin B12, calcium, magnesium, and potassium. Let me break down why each of these matters and what happens when you don't get enough.

Iron is essential for carrying oxygen in your blood. Low iron causes fatigue, weakness, and difficulty concentrating. Women are especially at risk for iron deficiency, particularly if they're still menstruating. If you're not eating much red meat or iron-rich plant foods like spinach and lentils, you might not be getting enough. Signs of low iron include feeling constantly tired despite adequate sleep, getting winded easily, and pale skin.

Vitamin D is crucial for bone health, immune function, and mood regulation. A lot of people are already deficient in vitamin D even before they start losing weight. When you're eating less and potentially spending less time outside because you have less energy, deficiency becomes even more likely. Low vitamin D can contribute to depression, muscle weakness, and increased risk of illness.

Vitamin B12 is needed for nerve function and red blood cell production. If you're not eating much meat, fish, eggs, or dairy, you might be low in B12. Deficiency causes fatigue, weakness, numbness or tingling in hands and feet, and cognitive issues like brain fog. This is especially important to watch if you're eating a mostly plant-based diet.

Calcium is obviously important for bones, but it's also involved in muscle function and nerve signaling. If you're not consuming dairy products or calcium-fortified alternatives, and you're eating less overall, you might not be getting enough. This is a long-term concern because low calcium intake over time increases your risk of osteoporosis.

Magnesium is involved in hundreds of biochemical reactions in your body. It helps with muscle and nerve function, blood sugar control, and blood pressure regulation. Low magnesium can cause muscle cramps, fatigue, irregular heartbeat, and difficulty sleeping. A lot of people are borderline deficient even on a normal diet.

Potassium is essential for heart function and muscle contractions. It also helps balance sodium levels and manage blood pressure. If you're not eating much fruit, vegetables, or potatoes, you might not be getting enough. Low potassium can cause muscle weakness, cramps, irregular heartbeat, and fatigue.

The solution is twofold. First, prioritize nutrient-dense foods when you do eat. Focus on getting the most nutritional bang for your buck. Second, consider supplementation to fill gaps. We'll talk about specific supplements later in this chapter.

Fiber and Gut Health on Reduced Food Intake

Here's something that doesn't get enough attention. When you're eating less food, you're almost certainly eating less fiber. And that can create problems.

Fiber is important for digestive health, blood sugar control, cholesterol management, and feeding the beneficial bacteria in your gut. Most people should be getting 25 to 35 grams of fiber per day. But when you're on a GLP-1 medication and eating small amounts, you might be getting half that or less.

Low fiber intake can lead to constipation, which is already a common side effect of GLP-1 medications. The combination of slow digestion from the medication plus low fiber can make constipation pretty miserable. It can also affect your gut microbiome, which plays a role in everything from immunity to mood to metabolism.

The challenge is that high-fiber foods tend to be filling. Raw vegetables, whole grains, beans, fruit. These are all foods that take up a lot of space in your stomach. When your appetite is suppressed and you can only eat small amounts, filling up on fiber-rich foods might mean you don't have room for adequate protein.

So you need to be strategic. Choose fiber sources that don't take up too much volume. Berries are great because they're relatively high in fiber but don't fill you up as much as something like a big salad. Chia seeds and ground flaxseed can be added to yogurt or protein shakes to boost fiber without adding much volume. Well-cooked vegetables are easier to eat in quantity than raw vegetables because cooking breaks down some of the fiber and reduces volume.

Psyllium husk is a fiber supplement that can help if you're struggling to get enough from food. It's particularly good for constipation. You can mix it into water or add it to smoothies. Start with a small amount and increase gradually to avoid bloating or gas.

Your gut microbiome also needs attention. The beneficial bacteria in your intestines thrive on fiber and a diverse range of plant foods. When you're eating less and your diet becomes less varied, your gut bacteria diversity can decline. This might affect digestion, immunity, and even how your body processes food.

Try to eat a variety of different plant foods even in small amounts. Different colors of fruits and vegetables contain different beneficial compounds. Even if you can only eat a few bites, having variety matters. Fermented foods like yogurt, kefir, sauerkraut, and kimchi can also support gut health by providing beneficial bacteria.

Meal Timing and Frequency: Finding What Works

There's a lot of debate about meal timing and frequency. Should you eat three meals a day? Six small meals? Intermittent fasting? The truth is, there's no one right answer. What matters is finding a pattern that helps you meet your protein and nutrient needs while feeling as good as possible.

On GLP-1 medications, a lot of people naturally drift toward eating less frequently. You might not be hungry for breakfast. You might skip lunch because you're still full from the day before. You end up eating once or twice a day just because that's all you can manage.

The problem with eating only once or twice a day is that it makes meeting your protein target really hard. If you need 120 grams of protein and you're only eating once, you'd have to consume all 120 grams in that one meal. Your body can only use so much protein at once for muscle building. Spreading protein across multiple meals is more effective.

A reasonable approach for most people is to aim for three smaller meals per day, even if they're very small. Each meal should include a good protein source. This gives you three opportunities to get protein in and makes it more manageable to hit your daily target.

If you genuinely can't handle three meals, at least try for two meals plus a protein shake or high-protein snack. The goal is to avoid having all your protein intake concentrated in a single eating window.

Meal timing relative to exercise can matter too. Having protein within a few hours after resistance training helps with muscle recovery and growth. You don't need to chug a protein shake the second you finish your workout, but getting protein in within two to three hours is beneficial.

Some people do well with intermittent fasting patterns on GLP-1 medications. For example, eating only during an eight-hour window each day. If this works for you and you can still meet your protein and nutrient needs, that's fine. But don't force yourself into a restrictive eating window if it means you're not getting adequate nutrition.

The best meal timing and frequency is the one you can stick with while meeting your nutritional needs. Experiment and see what feels sustainable.

Food Quality vs. Food Quantity

When you're focused on calories and portions, it's easy to forget that food quality matters too. Not all 1,500-calorie diets are created equal.

You could eat 1,500 calories of processed foods, sugary snacks, and low-nutrient meals and technically be in a calorie deficit. You'd lose some weight. But you'd probably feel terrible. Your energy would be low. Your hunger might be harder to control despite the medication. Your body composition wouldn't be as good. And your overall health wouldn't improve much.

Or you could eat 1,500 calories of whole foods, lean proteins, vegetables, fruits, and healthy fats. You'd lose weight, but you'd also feel better, have more stable energy, better nutrient status, and improved health markers.

Food quality affects how satisfied you feel, how well your body functions, and how sustainable your eating pattern is. Higher quality foods tend to be more nutrient-dense, meaning they provide more vitamins, minerals, and beneficial compounds per calorie.

This doesn't mean you have to eat perfectly all the time. You don't need to eliminate all processed foods or never have dessert. But the bulk of your diet should come from minimally processed, nutrient-dense sources.

Choose whole foods over processed foods when possible. A baked potato is better than potato chips. A piece of grilled chicken is better than chicken nuggets. Fresh fruit is better than fruit snacks. These swaps don't just affect nutrients. They often affect how your body processes the food and how satisfied you feel afterward.

When you do include treats or less nutritious foods, do it intentionally and in reasonable amounts. If you want ice cream, have some ice cream. Just don't let it become half your daily calories. Fit it in after you've hit your protein target and gotten some nutrient-dense foods in.

Anti-Inflammatory Eating Patterns

Chronic inflammation is linked to a whole host of health problems. Obesity, heart disease, diabetes, joint pain, autoimmune conditions. Losing weight reduces inflammation to some degree just by itself. But the types of foods you eat can either help reduce inflammation further or contribute to it.

An anti-inflammatory eating pattern emphasizes whole foods that have been shown to reduce inflammatory markers in the body. This isn't a specific diet. It's more of an approach to food choices.

Focus on foods high in omega-3 fatty acids. Fatty fish like salmon, mackerel, sardines, and trout are excellent sources. Walnuts, chia seeds, and flaxseeds also provide omega-3s, though in a different form that's not quite as potent. Omega-3s are among the most well-researched anti-inflammatory nutrients.

Include plenty of colorful fruits and vegetables. The pigments that give them their colors often have anti-inflammatory properties. Berries are particularly good. So are leafy greens, tomatoes, peppers, and cruciferous vegetables like broccoli and Brussels sprouts.

Use herbs and spices liberally. Turmeric, ginger, garlic, cinnamon, and many other spices have anti-inflammatory compounds. They also add flavor without adding calories, which is helpful when you're eating smaller portions.

Choose healthy fats. Olive oil, avocados, nuts, and seeds provide fats that don't promote inflammation the way some other fats do. Extra virgin olive oil in particular has been shown to have anti-inflammatory effects.

Limit foods that promote inflammation. These include highly processed foods, foods high in added sugars, refined carbohydrates like white bread and pastries, fried foods, and excessive amounts of red and processed meats. You don't have to eliminate these entirely, but keeping them as occasional choices rather than dietary staples is beneficial.

The Mediterranean diet is probably the best-studied anti-inflammatory eating pattern. It emphasizes fish, olive oil, vegetables, fruits, whole grains, legumes, and moderate amounts of wine. If you're looking for a framework to follow, Mediterranean-style eating is a solid choice that aligns well with weight loss goals.

Insulin Sensitivity and Food Choices

Insulin is the hormone that helps move glucose from your bloodstream into your cells. When your cells respond well to insulin, that's good insulin sensitivity. When they don't respond as well, that's insulin resistance.

Many people who struggle with weight have some degree of insulin resistance. GLP-1 medications help improve insulin sensitivity, which is one reason they work so well for weight loss and diabetes management. But your food choices can either support or undermine that improvement.

Foods that spike your blood sugar rapidly tend to make insulin resistance worse over time. These are mostly refined carbohydrates and added sugars. White bread, sugary drinks, candy, pastries, white rice, most breakfast cereals. When you eat these foods, your blood sugar shoots up quickly. Your pancreas has to pump out a lot of insulin to deal with it. Over time, this can make your cells less responsive to insulin.

Foods that release glucose more slowly into your bloodstream help maintain insulin sensitivity. These include whole grains, legumes, most vegetables, and foods that contain fiber, protein, and healthy fats along with carbohydrates.

When you're on a GLP-1 medication and trying to lose weight, prioritizing foods that support insulin sensitivity makes sense. It helps the medication work more effectively. It gives you more stable energy. It reduces cravings. And it improves your metabolic health long-term.

Practical strategies include pairing carbohydrates with protein or fat to slow digestion. If you're having rice, have it with chicken and vegetables, not by itself. If you're having fruit, pair it with some nuts or a bit of cheese. The protein and fat slow down how quickly the carbs hit your bloodstream.

Choose complex carbohydrates over simple ones most of the time. Sweet potatoes over white potatoes. Brown rice over white rice. Whole grain bread over white bread. Oats over sugary cereal. These swaps help keep blood sugar more stable.

And manage portion sizes of carbohydrates relative to your overall needs. You don't need to go low-carb unless you want to. But you also don't need massive portions of carbs at every meal. A moderate amount paired with good protein and vegetables is usually the sweet spot.

Supplements Worth Considering (And Ones to Skip)

Let's talk about supplementation. When you're eating less food and losing weight rapidly, certain supplements can be genuinely helpful. Others are a waste of money.

A basic multivitamin is a good insurance policy for most people on GLP-1 medications. It won't replace eating nutritious food, but it can help fill gaps. Look for one that provides a broad range of vitamins and minerals without megadoses of anything. You don't need 1,000% of the daily value for most nutrients.

Vitamin D is worth supplementing for most people, especially if you live in a northern climate or don't spend much time outside. Blood testing can tell you if you're deficient, but taking 1,000 to 2,000 IU per day is safe for most people and often beneficial.

Omega-3 supplements can be helpful if you're not eating fatty fish regularly. Look for a supplement that provides at least 500 to 1,000 mg of combined EPA and DHA, which are the active omega-3 fatty acids. Fish oil is the most common form, but algae-based omega-3s work too if you're vegetarian or don't like fish.

Magnesium supplementation can help if you're experiencing muscle cramps, poor sleep, or constipation. Magnesium citrate or glycinate are well-absorbed forms. Start with 200 to 400 mg per day. Too much magnesium can cause diarrhea, so start lower and increase if needed.

Fiber supplements like psyllium husk can be useful for managing constipation and ensuring you're getting adequate fiber when food intake is low.

Electrolyte supplements or beverages can be helpful if you're very active, sweating a lot, or dealing with side effects like vomiting or diarrhea that can deplete electrolytes. Look for options that provide sodium, potassium, and magnesium without a lot of added sugar.

Before adding protein supplements to your routine, talk with your doctor, especially if you have any kidney issues, digestive conditions, or other health concerns that might be affected by increased protein intake.

Now, supplements to skip. Fat burners and metabolism boosters are generally not worth it. Most of them don't work, and the ones that do have any effect are often stimulants that can make you feel jittery and anxious. You're already on a medication that's helping with weight loss. You don't need sketchy supplements on top of that.

Detox products and cleanses are unnecessary. Your liver and kidneys handle detoxification just fine. These products are usually expensive and don't do anything beneficial.

Appetite suppressants are pointless when you're on a GLP-1 medication. Your appetite is already suppressed. You don't need more suppression. In fact, you might need help eating enough, not eating less.

Expensive proprietary blends with long lists of exotic ingredients are usually overpriced and under-effective. Stick with well-researched individual supplements or simple formulations.

Working With a Registered Dietitian

If you're struggling to figure out your nutrition on GLP-1 medications, working with a registered dietitian can be incredibly valuable. Not a nutritionist or a health coach, but specifically a registered dietitian. That's someone with formal education and credentials in nutrition science.

A good dietitian can help you figure out how much you should be eating, create meal plans that meet your needs, identify nutrient deficiencies, manage side effects through food choices, and provide accountability and support.

They can be especially helpful if you have other health

conditions that complicate your nutrition needs. If you have diabetes, kidney disease, food allergies, digestive issues, or other medical conditions, a dietitian can help you navigate those challenges while optimizing your weight loss.

Many insurance plans cover dietitian visits, especially if you have diabetes or other medical conditions. If your insurance doesn't cover it, the out-of-pocket cost is usually reasonable for at least a few sessions. Even a single consultation can give you valuable insights and a plan to follow.

When choosing a dietitian, look for someone who has experience working with people on GLP-1 medications or at least experience with rapid weight loss scenarios. Not all dietitians are familiar with the specific challenges these medications create.

Be honest with your dietitian about what you're actually eating, not what you think you should be eating. They can't help you if they don't have accurate information. And don't be afraid to ask questions or speak up if something they recommend isn't working for you. Good dietitians want feedback and will adjust their recommendations based on your experience.

Nutritional optimization might seem like a minor detail compared to things like calorie deficit and protein intake. But when you're eating less food overall, making every bite count becomes more important. The quality and variety of what you eat affects how you feel, how well you function, and how successful you'll be long-term.

In the next chapter, we'll talk about metabolic factors and hormones that can affect your weight loss beyond just nutrition and exercise. If you've been doing everything right but still struggling, this is where we start looking deeper.

Chapter 9
The Metabolic Reset

A client came to me six months into her journey on tirzepatide. She'd done everything right. Tracked her food meticulously. Hit her protein targets every day. Exercised consistently. Got plenty of sleep. Managed stress. And yet, she'd only lost twelve pounds in six months. For someone her size, that was frustratingly slow.

We could have kept tweaking her diet and exercise, but at a certain point, you have to look deeper. We convinced her doctor to run a comprehensive metabolic panel. Turns out her thyroid was barely functioning. Once she started thyroid medication alongside her GLP-1, weight loss picked up dramatically. Within three months, she'd lost another twenty pounds.

This chapter is for people who've tried the basics and they're not working. Sometimes the issue isn't what you're eating or how much you're moving. Sometimes there's an underlying metabolic issue that's working against you.

When Basic Strategies Aren't Working

Before we dive into testing and medical interventions, let's make sure you've actually given the basics a fair shot.

Have you been tracking your food intake accurately for at least a month? Not guessing or estimating, but actually measuring and logging everything? Have you been hitting your protein targets consistently, not just occasionally? Have you been doing resistance training at least twice a week for at least two months? Have you been getting seven to nine hours of sleep most nights? Have you been managing stress reasonably well?

If the honest answer to any of those questions is no, then you need to tighten up the basics before assuming there's a metabolic issue. I see a lot of people jump straight to "something must be wrong with my hormones" when really they just haven't been consistent enough with the fundamentals.

But if you've been doing all of those things consistently for at least three months and your weight loss is still much slower than expected, or if you've been maintaining or even gaining weight despite being on a therapeutic dose of medication and following a solid plan, then it's time to look deeper.

Signs that there might be an underlying metabolic issue include losing less than 5% of your body weight after three months on a full dose, having severe fatigue that doesn't improve over time, experiencing hair loss beyond normal shedding, feeling cold all the time, having very dry skin, struggling with depression or mood issues, dealing with irregular periods or cycle changes, having persistent digestive issues, or seeing no improvement in health markers like blood sugar or cholesterol despite weight loss.

These symptoms don't automatically mean something is wrong. But they're worth investigating, especially if you're experiencing multiple symptoms at once.

Comprehensive Metabolic Testing (What to Ask Your Doctor For)

If you suspect an underlying issue, you need to get tested. You can't guess at what might be wrong. You need actual data.

Here's what you should ask your doctor to test. Not all of these will be necessary for everyone, but this is a comprehensive list of tests that can help identify metabolic barriers to weight loss.

Thyroid function is critical. Ask for a full thyroid panel, not just TSH. You want TSH, free T3, free T4, and thyroid antibodies. A lot of doctors will only test TSH, but that doesn't give you the whole picture. TSH can be normal even when your actual thyroid hormones are low. Free T3 and free T4 tell you what your active thyroid hormones are doing. Antibodies tell you if there's an autoimmune component affecting your thyroid.

Fasting insulin and fasting glucose tell you about insulin resistance. High fasting insulin even with normal glucose suggests insulin resistance. You can also ask for a hemoglobin A1C, which shows your average blood sugar over the past three months, and a HOMA-IR calculation, which estimates insulin resistance based on fasting glucose and insulin levels.

Cortisol can be checked through blood work, but timing matters because cortisol fluctuates throughout the day. A 24-hour urinary cortisol test gives a better picture of your overall cortisol levels. High cortisol can make weight loss extremely difficult.

Sex hormones matter too. For women, estrogen, progesterone, and testosterone levels can all affect weight. For men, testosterone is particularly important. Low testosterone in men makes it harder to build muscle and easier to gain fat. Hormone testing for women is best done at specific times in your cycle for accuracy, so discuss timing with your doctor.

DHEA-S is another hormone worth checking. It's produced by your adrenal glands and can indicate if there are issues with your stress hormone system.

Vitamin D, vitamin B12, iron, and ferritin should be checked because deficiencies in these can cause fatigue and other symptoms that mimic metabolic issues. They can also directly affect your metabolism.

Liver function tests and kidney function tests are good to have as baseline, especially if you're on multiple medications. These organs are crucial for metabolism and medication processing.

Cholesterol panel including HDL, LDL, and triglycerides gives you information about metabolic health. Sometimes these improve with weight loss, but sometimes they reveal underlying metabolic issues.

Your doctor might not want to order all of these tests at once. That's okay. Start with the most likely culprits based on your symptoms. Thyroid function, fasting insulin, and vitamin D are good starting points for most people.

Thyroid Function and GLP-1s

Your thyroid is a small gland in your neck that produces hormones regulating your metabolism. When your thyroid isn't working properly, weight loss becomes incredibly difficult, even with appetite suppression from GLP-1 medications.

Hypothyroidism, or low thyroid function, is more common than most people realize. Some estimates suggest that up to 10% of women and 5% of men have some degree of thyroid dysfunction, and many of them don't know it.

Symptoms of low thyroid function include unexplained weight gain or inability to lose weight, fatigue that doesn't improve with rest, feeling cold all the time especially in your hands and feet, dry skin and hair, hair loss or thinning, constipation, brain fog and difficulty concentrating, depression or mood changes, irregular or heavy periods for women, and muscle weakness.

If you have several of these symptoms and your weight loss

on GLP-1s has been minimal despite doing everything right, get your thyroid tested.

The relationship between thyroid function and GLP-1 medications is interesting. Some research suggests that rapid weight loss can temporarily lower thyroid hormones as your body tries to conserve energy. This is part of metabolic adaptation. For most people, this is mild and temporary. But if you already had borderline low thyroid function, rapid weight loss might push you into symptomatic hypothyroidism.

Treatment for hypothyroidism usually involves thyroid hormone replacement medication, most commonly levothyroxine. Once your thyroid levels are optimized, weight loss often becomes much easier. Your energy improves. You feel warmer. Your mood gets better. And the GLP-1 medication can work more effectively.

It's important to note that thyroid medication isn't a weight loss drug. It brings your thyroid function back to normal. If your thyroid is already functioning normally, taking thyroid medication won't help you lose weight and can actually be dangerous. Only take thyroid medication if testing confirms you actually need it.

Hormone Considerations: Cortisol, Testosterone, Estrogen

Let's talk about other hormones that can affect your weight loss response.

Cortisol is your primary stress hormone. It's essential for survival, but chronically elevated cortisol creates problems. High cortisol increases appetite, promotes fat storage especially around your midsection, breaks down muscle tissue, interferes with sleep, and promotes insulin resistance.

If you're under constant stress, not sleeping well, over-exercising, or dealing with certain medical conditions, your cortisol might be chronically elevated. This can absolutely interfere with weight loss even on GLP-1 medications.

Unfortunately, managing high cortisol often requires lifestyle changes rather than medication. Stress management techniques, adequate sleep, reducing or modifying intense exercise, and addressing sources of chronic stress are the main interventions. Sometimes therapy or counseling can help if stress is related to mental health or life circumstances.

In rare cases, very high cortisol is caused by a medical condition like Cushing's syndrome. That requires medical treatment. But for most people, cortisol issues are related to lifestyle and stress.

Testosterone matters for both men and women, though levels and effects differ. In men, low testosterone makes it harder to build and maintain muscle, increases fat storage, reduces energy and motivation, and can cause depression and brain fog. Men over 40 often experience gradual declines in testosterone, which can make weight loss harder.

Testosterone replacement therapy can be helpful for men

with genuinely low testosterone levels confirmed by blood testing. But it's not appropriate for everyone and should be prescribed and monitored by a doctor who understands hormone therapy.

Women also produce testosterone, just in smaller amounts. Low testosterone in women can cause similar issues with muscle mass and energy. High testosterone in women, often associated with PCOS, creates different problems we'll discuss in the next section.

Estrogen and progesterone affect weight, metabolism, and body composition in women. Estrogen levels naturally decline during menopause, which often coincides with weight gain and changes in where fat is stored. Lower estrogen can reduce metabolic rate and promote fat storage around the midsection.

Progesterone helps balance estrogen and affects water retention, mood, and sleep. Imbalances between estrogen and progesterone can contribute to weight issues, particularly in perimenopause.

Hormone replacement therapy during menopause can help some women, but it's a complex decision that depends on individual health history and risk factors. Discuss it thoroughly with your doctor if you're dealing with menopausal symptoms and struggling with weight loss.

Insulin Resistance: The Hidden Barrier

We touched on insulin sensitivity in the last chapter, but let's go deeper because insulin resistance is one of the most common metabolic barriers to weight loss.

Insulin resistance means your cells don't respond well to insulin. Your pancreas has to produce more and more insulin to get glucose into your cells. Over time, this leads to chronically high insulin levels even when your blood sugar looks normal.

High insulin levels make weight loss really hard because insulin is a storage hormone. When insulin is elevated, your body is in storage mode, not burning mode. It's actively trying to store fat rather than release it for energy.

Many people with significant weight to lose have some degree of insulin resistance. It's not always obvious because blood sugar might still be in the normal range. But fasting insulin levels tell the real story. If your fasting insulin is above 10 to 12 uIU/mL, you likely have insulin resistance even if your glucose is normal.

GLP-1 medications actually help improve insulin sensitivity, which is part of why they work so well. But if your insulin resistance is severe, the medication alone might not be enough. You might need to be more aggressive with dietary strategies that directly address insulin resistance.

Strategies that help improve insulin resistance include reducing refined carbohydrates and added sugars significantly, eating protein and fat with carbohydrates to slow glucose absorption, including regular physical activity especially resistance training, losing weight even small amounts, getting adequate sleep, managing stress, and in some cases, adding medications like metformin that directly improve insulin sensitivity.

If testing reveals significant insulin resistance, talk to your doctor about whether adding metformin or another insulin-sensitizing medication makes sense alongside your GLP-1 medication. The combination can be very effective for some people.

PCOS, Menopause, and Other Complicating Factors

Certain conditions make weight loss harder even under the best circumstances. Understanding how they interact with GLP-1 medications helps you set realistic expectations and develop better strategies.

PCOS, or polycystic ovary syndrome, affects about 10% of women of reproductive age. It involves hormone imbalances, particularly elevated testosterone and insulin resistance. Women with PCOS often struggle significantly with weight, and losing weight with PCOS is notoriously difficult.

GLP-1 medications can be particularly helpful for women with PCOS because they address the insulin resistance component. But weight loss might still be slower than for women without PCOS. You might need to be more careful with carbohydrate intake. You might need to exercise more consistently. And you might need additional medications to manage other aspects of PCOS.

If you have PCOS and you're on a GLP-1 medication, work closely with your doctor, ideally an endocrinologist who specializes in PCOS. Metformin is often prescribed alongside GLP-1 medications for women with PCOS. Birth control pills or other hormone medications might also be part of your treatment plan.

Menopause and perimenopause create hormonal shifts that make weight loss harder. Declining estrogen changes where fat is stored and can slow metabolism. Sleep disruptions from hot flashes and night sweats affect cortisol and appetite hormones. Mood changes can affect motivation and eating behaviors.

GLP-1 medications can definitely work during and after menopause, but results might be slower than for younger women. Hormone replacement therapy can help some women, but that's a decision to make with your doctor based on your health history.

Hashimoto's thyroiditis is an autoimmune condition affecting the thyroid. Even with thyroid medication, some people with Hashimoto's struggle with weight. GLP-1 medications can help, but managing the autoimmune component through diet and lifestyle is also important for some people.

Lipedema is a condition involving abnormal fat accumulation, usually in the legs and sometimes arms. It's often misdiagnosed as regular obesity, but it doesn't respond well to diet and exercise. GLP-1 medications can help with weight loss in unaffected areas but don't typically improve lipedema fat. If you have disproportionate fat accumulation that doesn't respond to anything, talk to your doctor about whether lipedema might be a factor.

Medication Interactions That Might Interfere

Some medications can interfere with weight loss even when you're doing everything right. If you're on any of these medications and struggling to lose weight, discuss alternatives with your doctor.

Certain antidepressants, particularly mirtazapine, paroxetine, and some tricyclic antidepressants, are associated with weight gain and can make weight loss harder. If you're on one of these and struggling, ask your doctor about switching to a more weight-neutral option like bupropion or sertraline.

Many antipsychotic medications cause significant weight gain. Olanzapine and clozapine are among the worst offenders, but others can affect weight too. These medications are often necessary for serious mental health conditions, so stopping them isn't always an option. But sometimes doses can be reduced or alternative medications tried.

Mood stabilizers like lithium and valproate can promote weight gain. If you're on these medications for bipolar disorder or other conditions, discuss with your psychiatrist whether alternatives exist or whether strategies can be implemented to minimize weight effects.

Steroids like prednisone cause weight gain and increase appetite. If you're on steroids long-term for conditions like autoimmune diseases, this can significantly interfere with weight loss. Work with your doctor to use the lowest effective dose and explore steroid-sparing alternatives when possible.

Beta blockers used for high blood pressure can slow metabolism slightly and make weight loss harder. If you're on a beta blocker and struggling, ask your doctor about switching to a different blood pressure medication that doesn't affect weight.

Birth control pills can affect weight in some women, though the effect is usually modest. If you started a new birth control around the same time weight loss stalled, it might be worth trying a different formulation or method.

Some diabetes medications besides GLP-1s can affect weight. Insulin and sulfonylureas can promote weight gain. Metformin is weight-neutral or slightly helps with weight loss. SGLT2 inhibitors can help with weight loss. If you're on multiple diabetes medications, discuss with your doctor whether your combination might be working against your weight loss goals.

Never stop or change medications on your own. Always discuss concerns with your doctor. Often there are alternatives that treat your condition effectively without interfering with weight loss.

When to Consider Metabolic Specialist Consultation

If you've tried everything in this book, you've been consistent for months, you've addressed the basics, and you're still not getting results, it might be time to see a specialist.

An endocrinologist specializes in hormones and metabolism. They can do more comprehensive testing than a primary care doctor and are better equipped to identify and treat complex metabolic issues. They can manage conditions like thyroid disease, PCOS, diabetes, and hormone imbalances.

If you have multiple metabolic issues or complex health conditions, an endocrinologist is the right specialist to coordinate your care. They can also work with your primary care doctor and other specialists to ensure all your medications and treatments are working together rather than against each other.

A registered dietitian who specializes in metabolic conditions can be invaluable. They understand how different conditions affect nutritional needs and can create eating plans that work with your metabolism rather than against it.

For women dealing with hormonal issues, a gynecologist or a doctor specializing in women's health and hormones can be helpful. They understand the connections between reproductive hormones, metabolism, and weight.

Some obesity medicine specialists focus specifically on

treating obesity as a complex medical condition. They're often up to date on the latest medications and treatment approaches and can provide comprehensive obesity treatment.

Signs you should consider specialist consultation include losing less than 2% of your body weight after six months on a therapeutic dose despite being compliant, having multiple symptoms suggesting metabolic issues, dealing with several medical conditions that complicate weight loss, taking multiple medications that might be interfering, or feeling like your primary care doctor isn't sure what else to try.

Getting a specialist referral usually requires going through your primary care doctor first. Explain your situation, share your food and exercise logs, and express that you feel like there might be underlying issues that need investigation. Most doctors will be supportive of referring you to a specialist if you've genuinely tried the basics and aren't seeing results.

Metabolic issues can be frustrating because they're invisible and often take time to diagnose. But once identified, they're usually treatable. Don't give up if the basics aren't working. Keep advocating for yourself until you get answers.

In the next chapter, we'll talk about lifestyle factors beyond diet and exercise that can affect your results. Things like sleep, stress, and daily habits that might be holding you back without.

Chapter 10
Lifestyle Factors You're Overlooking

A client was doing everything right on paper. Her food tracking was perfect. She hit her protein targets every day. She exercised regularly. She was on a good dose of semaglutide. But her weight loss had crawled to a near halt after the first two months.

When we dug deeper into her daily life, the issues became clear. She was sleeping four to five hours a night because of work stress. She was having two or three glasses of wine every evening to unwind. And she was so stressed that her cortisol levels were probably through the roof. Once we addressed those lifestyle factors, her weight loss picked back up within a few weeks.

This chapter is about all the things outside of food and exercise that can make or break your results. These factors don't always get the attention they deserve, but they matter more than most people realize.

Sleep: The Underrated Weight Loss Tool

If you're not sleeping enough, you're making weight loss significantly harder. It's that simple.

When you don't get adequate sleep, your body produces more ghrelin, the hormone that stimulates hunger, and less leptin, the hormone that signals fullness. GLP-1 medications help counteract this to some degree, but they don't completely override the effects of sleep deprivation. You might find yourself hungrier and less satisfied even with the medication working.

Poor sleep also increases cortisol, which we talked about in the last chapter. Elevated cortisol promotes fat storage, particularly around your midsection. It increases insulin resistance. It makes you crave high-calorie comfort foods. All of that works against weight loss.

Sleep deprivation affects your decision-making and willpower. When you're exhausted, you're more likely to skip workouts, make poor food choices, and give in to cravings. You're also more likely to eat for energy rather than hunger. Your brain is looking for quick energy sources, which usually means sugar and refined carbs.

Beyond weight loss, inadequate sleep affects muscle recovery, immune function, mood, cognitive performance, and overall health. If you're exercising regularly but not sleeping enough, you're not getting the full benefits of that exercise because your body doesn't have time to recover and adapt.

Most adults need seven to nine hours of sleep per night. Not six. Not five. Seven to nine. If you're consistently getting less than that, improving your sleep should be a top priority.

Here's how to improve your sleep. Keep a consistent sleep schedule, going to bed and waking up at roughly the same time every day, even on weekends. Your body thrives on routine.

Make your bedroom conducive to sleep. Keep it cool, ideally between 60 and 67 degrees Fahrenheit. Make it as dark as possible with blackout curtains or an eye mask. Minimize noise or use a white noise machine. Your bedroom should be a sleep sanctuary, not a multipurpose room.

Avoid screens for at least an hour before bed. The blue light from phones, tablets, and computers interferes with melatonin production, making it harder to fall asleep. If you must use screens, use blue light filters or glasses.

Limit caffeine after early afternoon. Caffeine has a half-life of about five to six hours, meaning half of it is still in your system that long after you consume it. If you have coffee at 3 PM, a significant amount of caffeine is still affecting you at 9 PM.

Avoid alcohol close to bedtime. We'll talk more about alcohol shortly, but it's worth noting here that while alcohol might help you fall asleep initially, it disrupts sleep quality later in the night. You wake up more often and spend less time in deep, restorative sleep.

Create a wind-down routine. Do calming activities in the hour before bed. Read, take a warm bath, do gentle stretching, practice meditation or deep breathing. Signal to your body that it's time to transition to sleep.

If you struggle with insomnia or sleep disorders like sleep apnea, talk to your doctor. These conditions need proper treatment. Sleep apnea in particular is common in people who are overweight and can significantly interfere with weight loss. Getting it treated can make a huge difference.

Stress Management and Weight Loss Resistance

Chronic stress is one of the most overlooked barriers to weight loss. You can have perfect nutrition and exercise, but if your stress levels are constantly elevated, you're fighting an uphill battle.

We've already talked about cortisol, the primary stress hormone. When you're stressed, your body perceives a threat and responds by conserving energy and storing fat. This made sense evolutionarily when stress usually meant physical danger or scarcity. But in modern life, stress is usually psychological and chronic, not physical and temporary.

High cortisol increases appetite, particularly for high-calorie, high-sugar foods. It promotes fat storage around your abdomen. It breaks down muscle tissue for energy. It interferes with sleep. It reduces insulin sensitivity. All of this makes weight loss harder.

Stress also affects behavior in ways that sabotage weight loss. When you're stressed, you're more likely to skip workouts, eat emotionally, make impulsive food choices, and abandon healthy habits. You're also more likely to use food as a coping mechanism.

GLP-1 medications don't reduce stress or lower cortisol. They suppress physical hunger, but they don't address stress-driven eating or the metabolic effects of chronic stress. If stress is a major factor in your life, you need to address it directly.

Strategies for managing stress include regular exercise, which is one of the most effective stress reducers. Even a 20-minute walk can lower cortisol levels significantly.

Meditation and mindfulness practices have been shown to reduce stress and lower cortisol. Even just a few minutes a day can help. Apps like Headspace, Calm, or Insight Timer can guide you if you're new to meditation.

Deep breathing exercises are simple but effective. When you're feeling stressed, take five minutes to breathe slowly and deeply. This activates your parasympathetic nervous system, which calms your body's stress response.

Social connection and support help buffer stress. Spending time with friends and family, talking about what's bothering you, and feeling connected to others all reduce stress.

Therapy or counseling can be invaluable if you're dealing with significant stress, anxiety, or trauma. A good therapist can help you develop coping strategies and address underlying issues contributing to stress.

Time management and boundaries help reduce chronic stress from overcommitment. Learning to say no, delegating tasks, and creating space in your schedule for rest and recovery can make a big difference.

Hobbies and activities you enjoy provide stress relief and give you something to focus on besides work and obligations. Whether it's reading, gardening, playing music, or anything else that brings you joy, make time for it.

You can't eliminate stress entirely. Life is stressful sometimes. But you can develop better tools for managing it so it doesn't completely derail your health and weight loss goals.

Alcohol: The Progress Killer

Let's talk about alcohol because it's a bigger issue than most people realize, especially for weight loss.

Alcohol contains seven calories per gram, which is almost as much as fat at nine calories per gram. Those calories add up quickly. A glass of wine has about 120 to 150 calories. A beer has 150 to 200 calories. Mixed drinks can easily be 200 to 400 calories depending on what's in them. If you're having two or three drinks several times a week, that's potentially 1,000 to 2,000 calories per week that might not be registering as food in your mind.

But alcohol's effects on weight loss go beyond just

calories. When you consume alcohol, your body prioritizes metabolizing it over everything else. While your liver is processing alcohol, it's not burning fat. Fat burning essentially stops until the alcohol is cleared from your system. This can last for hours after drinking.

Alcohol also lowers inhibitions and impairs decision-making. You're more likely to overeat when you've been drinking. The late-night pizza or snacks that happen after a few drinks can easily add several hundred more calories beyond the alcohol itself.

Alcohol disrupts sleep quality. You might fall asleep more easily after drinking, but your sleep is less restorative. You spend less time in deep sleep and REM sleep. You're more likely to wake up during the night. Poor sleep then affects hunger hormones, energy levels, and decision-making the next day.

Alcohol can increase appetite and cravings, even with GLP-1 medication on board. Some people find that the appetite suppression from their medication is less effective on days when they drink.

Regular alcohol consumption can affect liver function over time, which matters because your liver is crucial for metabolism and fat burning. It can also contribute to insulin resistance.

I'm not saying you can never have a drink. But if you're having alcohol regularly and your weight loss has stalled, reducing or eliminating alcohol for a few weeks might help you break through. Many people are surprised by how much difference it makes.

If you do choose to drink, do it mindfully. Decide in advance how much you'll have. Choose lower-calorie options like wine or spirits with soda water instead of high-calorie mixed drinks. Make sure you've hit your protein target for the day before you drink. And limit frequency to special occasions rather than daily or near-daily drinking.

For some people, eliminating alcohol entirely during the active weight loss phase makes sense. You can reintroduce it in moderation later if you want. But while you're trying to lose weight, especially if progress has been slow, alcohol might be holding you back more than you realize.

Social Eating Patterns and Hidden Calories

Your social life and eating environment can significantly affect your results without you even noticing.

When you eat with other people, you tend to eat more. This is called social facilitation of eating. You match the pace and portion sizes of the people around you. If everyone at the table is having appetizers, entrees, and dessert, you're more likely to do the same. If your dining companions are eating quickly and having second helpings, you probably will too.

GLP-1 medications help with this to some degree because you physically can't eat as much. But you can still eat more than you need in social settings, especially if the food is really good or if you're distracted by conversation.

Restaurant meals are particularly challenging. Portions are often two to three times larger than what you'd serve yourself at home. Food is prepared with more butter, oil, and salt than you'd use in your own cooking. A restaurant meal can easily be 1,500 to 2,000 calories even if it doesn't seem excessive.

Social pressure to eat can be real. Family gatherings, work events, celebrations. There's often an expectation that you'll eat what's offered or join in with whatever everyone else is having. Declining food can feel awkward or lead to unwanted comments about your eating or weight loss.

Strategies for managing social eating include eating something protein-rich before social events so you're not starving when you arrive. This makes it easier to make good choices and eat reasonable portions.

In restaurants, ask for dressings and sauces on the side. Order grilled or baked proteins instead of fried. Skip the bread basket or ask the server not to bring it. Consider splitting an entree or immediately boxing half to take home before you start eating.

Be selective about which social eating occasions really matter. You don't have to indulge at every birthday party, work lunch, or casual gathering. Save the flexibility for events that are truly special to you.

Practice saying no without over-explaining. You don't owe

anyone an explanation for your food choices. A simple "No thank you, I'm good" is sufficient. If people push, you can say "I'm not hungry right now" or "Maybe later" and change the subject.

Focus on the social aspect of events rather than the food. Engage in conversation. Participate in activities. Enjoy the company. Food doesn't have to be the centerpiece of every social interaction.

Emotional Eating on GLP-1s (Yes, It's Still Possible)

One of the most interesting things about GLP-1 medications is that they suppress physical hunger really effectively, but they don't necessarily address emotional or psychological drivers of eating.

Physical hunger is that stomach-growling, low-energy, genuinely-need-food feeling. GLP-1 medications reduce or eliminate this for most people. But emotional eating is different. It's eating in response to feelings rather than physical hunger. Stress, boredom, loneliness, anxiety, sadness, even happiness can trigger eating.

A lot of people discover that once physical hunger is taken out of the equation, they realize how much of their eating was driven by emotions. They're not hungry, but they still want to eat when they're stressed. They still think about food when they're bored. They still crave certain foods when they're sad.

The medication makes it easier not to eat in these situations because you're not physically hungry. But the urge might still be there. And if you consistently give in to emotional eating, even in smaller amounts than before, it can slow your progress.

Signs that you might be eating emotionally include eating when you're not physically hungry, eating in response to specific emotions or situations, eating quickly without really tasting food, eating while doing something else like watching TV or working, feeling guilty or ashamed after eating, or using food as a reward or comfort.

Addressing emotional eating requires identifying your triggers. What situations or emotions lead you to want food? Once you know your triggers, you can develop alternative coping strategies.

If you eat when you're stressed, find other stress-relief methods. Go for a walk, call a friend, do deep breathing, take a bath. If you eat when you're bored, find engaging activities that occupy your hands and mind. If you eat when you're sad, allow yourself to feel the sadness rather than suppressing it with food. Talk to someone, journal, or engage in a comforting activity that isn't eating.

Sometimes emotional eating is deeply ingrained and tied to childhood experiences, trauma, or mental health issues. If you're struggling with this, working with a therapist who specializes in eating behaviors can be really helpful. Cognitive behavioral therapy and dialectical behavior therapy are particularly effective for addressing emotional eating.

Remember, GLP-1 medications are powerful tools, but they're not a cure for emotional or psychological relationships with food. That work still needs to happen, just without the added burden of constant physical hunger.

Environmental Factors: Temperature, Light Exposure

Here are some factors that most people never think about, but they can affect your metabolism and weight loss.

Temperature exposure, particularly cold exposure, can increase calorie burning. When you're cold, your body has to work to maintain its core temperature, which burns calories. This is called thermogenesis. Some research suggests that spending time in cooler temperatures or taking cold showers can slightly boost metabolism.

This doesn't mean you should freeze yourself, but keeping your home a bit cooler, especially at night, might have a small beneficial effect. Sleeping in a cool room improves sleep quality anyway, which has bigger weight loss benefits than the thermogenesis effect.

Light exposure affects your circadian rhythm, which influences metabolism, hunger hormones, and sleep. Getting bright light exposure, especially natural sunlight, early in the day helps regulate your circadian rhythm. This can improve sleep quality at night and help regulate appetite hormones during the day.

Conversely, exposure to bright light late at night, especially blue light from screens, disrupts your circadian rhythm and can interfere with sleep and metabolism. We talked about this in the sleep section, but it's worth emphasizing. Your light exposure patterns throughout the day matter for more than just sleep.

Standing and moving throughout the day, which we discussed as NEAT in an earlier chapter, is also an environmental factor. If your environment requires you to move, you'll burn more calories. Setting up your workspace to require standing or movement can help. Taking stairs instead of elevators. Parking farther away. These environmental choices add up.

The food environment in your home matters too. If your kitchen is stocked with tempting high-calorie foods, you'll be more likely to eat them even with appetite suppression. If you have to go to the store to get treats, you're less likely to eat them on impulse. Controlling your food environment is one of the easiest ways to support your goals.

Medication Timing Optimization

When you take your GLP-1 medication can affect how you tolerate it and potentially how well it works.

Most GLP-1 medications are taken once weekly. You can take them at any time of day, but consistency helps. Pick a day and time that works with your schedule and stick with it.

Some people prefer taking their injection in the evening so

any initial side effects like nausea happen while they're sleeping. Others prefer morning injections so they can monitor how they feel during the day. There's no right answer. It's about what works best for you.

If you experience increased nausea or fatigue in the day or two after your injection, you might want to schedule your injection before days when you don't have major obligations. Injecting on Friday evening means the worst of the side effects happen over the weekend when you have more flexibility.

The injection site can affect absorption slightly. Abdomen tends to have the most consistent absorption. Thighs absorb slightly more slowly. Arms can work but are harder to self-inject. Rotating sites helps prevent tissue changes, but you can also rotate within the same general area. This week's injection goes on the left side of your abdomen, next week on the right side, and so on.

Room temperature medication is more comfortable to inject than cold medication. If you keep your medication in the refrigerator, take it out 30 minutes before injecting to let it warm up slightly.

Make sure you're injecting into subcutaneous fat, not muscle. Pinching the skin before inserting the needle helps ensure you're getting the fat layer. If you're very lean, you might need to pinch more firmly or use a shorter needle.

Building Sustainable Habits

All of these lifestyle factors matter, but trying to change everything at once is overwhelming and usually doesn't work. Sustainable change happens gradually.

Pick one or two areas to focus on first. Maybe sleep is your biggest issue. Focus on improving sleep for a few weeks before adding anything else. Once better sleep feels like a normal part of your routine, tackle the next thing.

Stack new habits onto existing routines. If you want to start meditating, do it right after you brush your teeth in the morning. Your tooth-brushing habit serves as a trigger for the meditation habit. If you want to drink more water, drink a glass every time you take your medication. The medication becomes the cue for hydration.

Make habits as easy as possible to do. If you want to exercise in the morning, lay out your workout clothes the night before. If you want to eat more vegetables, buy pre-cut vegetables so preparation is minimal. Remove barriers that make good habits harder to do.

Track your habits in some way. This could be a simple checklist, an app, or just mentally noting whether you did the thing. Tracking creates accountability and helps you see patterns over time.

Be patient with yourself. You won't be perfect. You'll have days or weeks where you slip. That's normal. What matters is getting back on track, not being flawless.

Focus on what you can control. You can't control your genetics, your age, or your metabolic rate. You can control your habits, your food choices, your movement, your sleep, and your stress management. Put your energy into the things you can actually influence.

Celebrate small wins. You slept eight hours three nights this week? That's progress. You chose water instead of wine at dinner? That's a win. You went for a walk even though you didn't feel like it? That counts. Acknowledging these victories keeps you motivated.

Lifestyle factors often get dismissed as minor details compared to diet and exercise. But they're not minor. They're the foundation that everything else is built on. You can have perfect nutrition and great workouts, but if you're sleep-deprived, chronically stressed, drinking regularly, and eating emotionally, your progress will suffer.

These factors are worth your attention. They're worth addressing. And often, fixing lifestyle issues is what finally unlocks the results you've been working toward.

In the next section of the book, we'll move into special situations. Things like losing the last ten pounds, dealing with weight regain, and considerations for specific populations. But make sure you've got these lifestyle factors handled first. They affect everyone, regardless of your specific situation.

PART 4

Special Situations

Chapter 11
The Last 10-20 Pounds

A client who'd lost sixty pounds came to me frustrated and defeated. She'd been stuck at the same weight for three months. She wanted to lose another fifteen pounds to hit what she considered her ideal weight, but nothing was working. Her food was dialed in. She was exercising consistently. She'd increased her medication dose. Still, the scale wouldn't budge.

We had a hard conversation. I asked her why fifteen more pounds mattered. What would change if she lost that weight? She couldn't really articulate it beyond "I just thought I'd be thinner." When we looked at her body composition, she'd actually gained muscle over those three months while maintaining her weight. She looked leaner and more toned. Her clothes fit better. Her health markers were excellent.

Sometimes the last ten or twenty pounds aren't actually necessary. And when they are necessary, getting them off requires a completely different approach than the weight you lost earlier in your journey.

Why the Last Bit Is Always Hardest

There's a reason the saying exists: "The last ten pounds are the hardest." It's not just in your head. There are legitimate physiological reasons why weight loss gets progressively harder as you get leaner.

First, your body requires less energy at a lower weight. When you weighed fifty pounds more, your body needed significantly more calories just to maintain basic functions. Now that you're lighter, your calorie needs have dropped. What was a meaningful deficit six months ago might barely be a deficit anymore.

Second, your body fights harder to preserve remaining fat stores as you get leaner. When you had more fat to lose, your body was relatively willing to release it. But as you approach a lower body fat percentage, your body perceives this as a potential threat and activates stronger adaptive mechanisms to prevent further loss.

Leptin, the hormone that signals adequate energy stores, is produced by fat cells. As you lose fat, leptin levels drop. Lower leptin tells your brain that energy stores are insufficient, which triggers increased hunger and decreased metabolism. GLP-1 medications help override the hunger signal, but they don't prevent the metabolic slowdown.

Your body becomes more metabolically efficient as you lose weight. This is metabolic adaptation, which we've discussed before. But it becomes more pronounced the leaner you get.

Your body learns to function on fewer calories, burning less energy for the same activities.

You're also likely closer to your body's natural set point. Your body has a weight range it's comfortable maintaining based on your genetics, history, and biology. As you approach or go below that set point, your body resists further weight loss more aggressively.

And finally, the margin for error gets smaller. When you had a lot of weight to lose, you could have imperfect tracking, occasional overeating, and still see progress because your deficit was large. Now, every extra 100 calories matters. A slightly too generous portion here, an untracked snack there, and your small deficit disappears.

Adjusting Expectations for Goal Weight

Before you fight to lose those last ten or twenty pounds, take a step back and honestly evaluate whether you need to lose them.

The number you have in your head as your goal weight might not be realistic or necessary for your body. That number might be based on what you weighed in high school, what a chart says you should weigh, what a friend weighs, or just an arbitrary number that sounds good.

But your body at forty-five years old isn't the same as your body at eighteen. You have different muscle mass, different bone density, different hormone levels. Trying to achieve or maintain a weight that was natural for you as a teenager might not be sustainable or healthy now.

BMI charts can be misleading too. They don't account for muscle mass, bone structure, or body composition. Someone who lifts weights regularly might have a higher BMI because muscle weighs more than fat, but they're healthier and leaner than someone with a lower BMI who has less muscle.

Ask yourself some hard questions. Are you healthy at your current weight? Are your blood pressure, blood sugar, cholesterol, and other health markers in good ranges? Do you feel good? Do you have energy? Can you do the activities you want to do? Are your clothes fitting the way you want?

If the answers to those questions are yes, then maybe you don't need to lose more weight. Maybe you need to focus on body recomposition, which we'll talk about shortly, rather than weight loss.

Consider whether the goal weight you're chasing is actually about health or if it's about aesthetics and perhaps unrealistic beauty standards. There's nothing wrong with wanting to look a certain way, but be honest about whether the pursuit is healthy and whether achieving it would actually make you happier.

Talk to your doctor about what weight range is healthy for you specifically, given your age, health history, and body composition. Their input might help you set more realistic and health-focused goals.

Body Recomposition vs. Scale Weight

This is where a lot of people get stuck. They're fixated on a number on the scale when what they really want is to look leaner, more toned, and more fit. Those things don't always correlate with lower scale weight.

Body recomposition means changing your body composition by losing fat and gaining or maintaining muscle without necessarily losing weight. You might stay the same weight or even gain a few pounds, but you look dramatically different because muscle is denser than fat.

This is especially relevant for people in the last ten or twenty pounds of their goal. At this point, losing more fat while building muscle is often a better strategy than just trying to lose more weight.

If you've been doing resistance training consistently, you might be building muscle while losing fat. The scale doesn't move, but you're getting smaller because muscle takes up less space than fat. Your clothes fit better. You look more defined. But the scale is lying to you by staying the same.

This is why body composition measurements or progress photos are so much more valuable than scale weight at this stage. Measure your waist, hips, thighs, and arms. Take photos from the front, side, and back every few weeks. Pay attention to how your clothes fit. These indicators tell you more about your progress than the scale does.

If body recomposition is your goal, you need to prioritize

resistance training and adequate protein even more than you have been. You might need to eat at maintenance calories or even a slight surplus to support muscle growth. You definitely need to be patient because recomposition is slower than straight weight loss.

Some people find that they look better and feel better at a slightly higher weight with more muscle than they would at a lower weight with less muscle. A person who weighs 150 pounds with good muscle mass looks leaner and more toned than someone who weighs 140 pounds with poor muscle mass.

The point is, don't let the scale dictate your success at this stage. Use multiple measures to evaluate progress, and be open to the possibility that your body looks and feels its best at a weight that's higher than you originally planned.

Maintenance Strategies

At some point, whether you've lost all the weight you wanted or you've decided you're happy where you are, you need to shift from active weight loss to maintenance. This transition can be tricky.

Maintenance doesn't mean going back to eating however you want. It means finding a sustainable way of eating that allows you to maintain your current weight without being overly restrictive.

If you've been in a deficit for months, your metabolism has

adapted. You can't just suddenly increase your calories back to what they theoretically should be for your weight. You'll likely gain weight if you do that.

A gradual approach works better. Increase your calories by 100 to 200 per week for several weeks until you reach a level where your weight stabilizes. This gives your metabolism time to recover and helps you figure out your actual maintenance calories through trial and error.

During this process, keep tracking your food and weighing yourself regularly. You're trying to find the sweet spot where you're eating enough to feel satisfied and energized but not so much that you start regaining weight.

You might find that you need to stay on your GLP-1 medication to maintain your weight. That's completely fine and actually quite common. A lot of people need the appetite suppression from the medication to maintain their weight loss long-term. That doesn't mean you failed. It means you're using the tool available to you to sustain your results.

If you want to try maintaining without the medication, discuss with your doctor about gradually reducing your dose while carefully monitoring your weight and appetite. Some people can transition off successfully. Others find that their appetite returns too strongly and weight starts creeping back up. There's no shame in staying on the medication indefinitely if that's what works for you.

Maintenance also requires continuing the habits that got

you here. You still need to prioritize protein. You still need to exercise regularly, especially resistance training. You still need adequate sleep and stress management. The only thing that changes is you're eating a bit more than you were during active weight loss.

When to Consider Transitioning Off GLP-1s

This is a personal decision that should be made with your doctor's guidance. There's no rule that says you have to stop taking these medications once you reach your goal weight.

Some people choose to stay on them indefinitely because the appetite suppression helps them maintain their weight loss. Research on long-term use is still developing, but so far, staying on these medications long-term appears to be safe for most people.

Other people want to try maintaining without medication because of cost, side effects, or personal preference. That's a valid choice too.

If you're considering stopping the medication, do it gradually under medical supervision. Don't just stop cold turkey. Your doctor might recommend slowly decreasing your dose over several weeks or months to see how your appetite and weight respond.

Be prepared for your appetite to return. This is normal and expected. The medication was suppressing your natural hunger signals. When you stop taking it, those signals come back. You'll need to rely more heavily on habits, portion control, and food choices to manage your eating.

Some people find that after losing weight and maintaining it for a while, their appetite and hunger cues are more normalized than they were before. They don't feel ravenously hungry all the time like they did before starting the medication. But they do feel more hunger than they did while on the medication.

Watch your weight closely after stopping. Weigh yourself at least weekly. If you start regaining weight, that's useful information. You can make adjustments to your eating and exercise, or you can discuss with your doctor about restarting the medication before significant regain happens.

There's also the option of staying on a lower maintenance dose rather than stopping completely. Some people do well on the lowest dose just to keep appetite in check without needing the full therapeutic dose. This can be a good middle ground.

The decision about whether and when to stop should be based on your individual situation, how you're feeling, whether you can afford to continue, and what your doctor recommends. There's no right or wrong answer. Do what works for you.

Psychological Adjustment to New Body Size

Here's something that doesn't get talked about enough. Losing a significant amount of weight changes how you look, but it doesn't always immediately change how you see yourself or how you feel about your body.

A lot of people expect to feel completely different once they hit their goal weight. They expect to feel confident, happy, and totally satisfied with their appearance. Sometimes that happens. But often, people are surprised to find that they still have complicated feelings about their bodies even after losing weight.

You might look in the mirror and still see your old body. This is called phantom fat. Your brain hasn't caught up with the reality of your new size. You reach for clothes in your old size. You're surprised when you fit through spaces that used to be tight. It takes time for your self-perception to adjust.

You might also find that losing weight didn't solve all the problems you thought it would solve. If you had relationship issues, career frustrations, or general unhappiness before, losing weight doesn't magically fix those things. Weight loss can improve your health and energy, but it's not a cure for life's other challenges.

Some people experience grief or loss after significant weight loss. Your body was part of your identity for a long time. Letting go of that identity, even though you wanted to change it, can be emotionally complicated. You might miss aspects of your old life or old self even while being happy about your progress.

Loose skin is a reality for many people who lose significant weight, especially if the loss was rapid or if you're older. Loose skin can be really hard to deal with emotionally. You worked so hard to lose weight, and now you're left with excess skin that makes you feel self-conscious. Compression clothing can help. Strength training can help build muscle that fills out some of the skin. Surgery is an option for severe cases. But mostly, it's about accepting that your body has been through a major transformation and it's okay if it doesn't look exactly like you imagined.

Relationships can change when you lose weight too. Some partners are supportive and encouraging. Others feel threatened or insecure. Friends or family members who also struggle with weight might treat you differently. You might get attention or comments about your body that feel uncomfortable even when they're meant as compliments.

All of these psychological and social adjustments are normal. If you're struggling, consider talking to a therapist who specializes in body image or eating issues. Having support during this transition can make a huge difference.

Remember that your worth isn't determined by your weight or appearance. Losing weight is an accomplishment, and you should feel proud of the work you've done. But you were a valuable person before you lost weight, and you're a valuable person now. Your body size doesn't define you.

Moving Forward

The last ten or twenty pounds can feel like the hardest

part of the journey. And in many ways, they are. But they're also an opportunity to refine your approach, focus on body composition rather than just scale weight, and figure out what maintenance will look like for you.

Be patient with yourself. Be realistic about your goals. And be willing to adjust your expectations if you find that your body is happy and healthy at a weight that's higher than what you originally planned.

Sometimes the journey doesn't end where you thought it would. And that's okay. What matters is that you've improved your health, built sustainable habits, and created a life that feels good in your body. The exact number on the scale is far less important than how you feel and how you're able to live your life.

In the next chapter, we'll talk about what to do if you start regaining weight after having success. Weight regain is common, but it's not inevitable, and there are strategies for addressing it before it becomes significant.

Chapter 12
Regaining After Initial Success

You lost thirty pounds. Maybe forty. Maybe more. The medication worked incredibly well. You felt great. Your clothes fit better. Your health markers improved. And then, slowly, the scale started creeping back up. Even though you're still taking your medication. Even though you haven't consciously changed anything.

This is one of the most frustrating experiences people have with GLP-1 medications. Weight regain while still on the medication feels confusing and demoralizing. But it happens, and understanding why it happens is the first step toward addressing it.

Why Some People Start Regaining on Medication

Weight regain while on GLP-1 medications isn't uncommon. Studies show that some people start regaining weight after six to twelve months, even while continuing their medication at the same dose.

This doesn't mean the medication stopped working entirely. It usually means that one or more factors have shifted in a way that's tipped the balance from weight loss or maintenance toward gradual weight gain.

Your appetite suppression might have lessened over time. The medication might not be suppressing your hunger as effectively as it did initially. You feel hungrier more often. Food seems more appealing. The constant feeling of fullness that made it easy to eat less has diminished somewhat.

Your activity level might have decreased without you fully realizing it. Maybe you're exercising less frequently or less intensely than you were during active weight loss. Maybe your daily movement has dropped. You're sitting more, walking less, generally moving your body less throughout the day.

Your food intake has likely increased, even if subtly. Portions have gotten slightly larger. You're snacking more often. You're having treats more frequently. The tight tracking and careful attention you paid to food in the beginning has relaxed. This is called diet creep, and we'll talk more about it shortly.

Your metabolism has adapted to your lower weight and reduced calorie intake. Your body is now more efficient at using energy, which means you burn fewer calories for the same activities. What used to create a deficit no longer does.

Stress, sleep, or other lifestyle factors might have changed. Maybe you went through a stressful period at work. Maybe your sleep has gotten worse. Maybe you started drinking more alcohol. Any of these can affect weight even when you're on medication.

Or there might be a medical factor at play. A new medication that affects weight. A change in hormone levels. An undiagnosed thyroid issue. Something that's working against the GLP-1 medication's effects.

The key is identifying which factors are contributing to your regain so you can address them specifically rather than just panicking and assuming the medication has stopped working.

Metabolic Adaptation Over Time

We've talked about metabolic adaptation several times in this book, but it's worth revisiting here because it plays a significant role in weight regain.

When you lose weight, your metabolism slows down. Part of this is expected. A smaller body requires fewer calories. But metabolic adaptation goes beyond that. Your body becomes more efficient at using energy, burning fewer calories than would be predicted for your new size.

This adaptation happens gradually over the course of weight loss. The longer you've been in a deficit and the more weight you've lost, the more pronounced the adaptation becomes.

At some point, the calorie level that was creating a nice deficit when you started might no longer be a deficit at all. You might actually be eating at or slightly above your adapted maintenance level, which would cause gradual weight regain.

If you lost weight eating 1,500 calories per day, you might find that six months later, eating 1,500 calories causes you to slowly gain weight because your metabolism has slowed and adapted. You might need to eat 1,300 or 1,400 calories to maintain, which is frustrating and feels unfair. Because it kind of is unfair.

This is why taking diet breaks during weight loss can be beneficial. They give your metabolism a chance to recover somewhat before continuing with further weight loss. If you didn't take breaks and you've been in a deficit for a long time, your metabolism might be quite suppressed.

The solution involves either accepting a higher calorie restriction than feels reasonable, working to reverse some of the metabolic adaptation through diet breaks or reverse dieting, or increasing your activity level to create a deficit without eating less. Or some combination of all three.

Medication Tolerance: Is It Real?

There's debate in the medical community about whether true tolerance to GLP-1 medications develops over time. Tolerance would mean that your body becomes less responsive to the medication's effects, requiring higher doses to achieve the same results.

Some research suggests that the effectiveness of GLP-1 medications can diminish slightly over time for some people.

The appetite suppression isn't as strong at twelve months as it was at three months, even on the same dose. But this isn't universal. Plenty of people maintain strong appetite suppression long-term.

What's likely happening for many people isn't true pharmacological tolerance, but rather a combination of factors. Your body adapting metabolically. Your behaviors drifting back toward old patterns. Psychological habituation to the medication where you're less mindful about eating because you're relying on the medication to do all the work.

It's also possible that your dose isn't high enough anymore. If you started on a lower dose and never increased, you might benefit from a higher dose now that your body has adapted. Or if you were doing well on a certain dose but have regained weight, increasing the dose might help, though that's a decision for your doctor to make.

Some people do seem to genuinely become less responsive to a specific GLP-1 medication over time. In those cases, switching to a different medication in the same class might help. Switching from semaglutide to tirzepatide, or vice versa, can sometimes produce renewed response. But again, that's something to discuss with your doctor, not a decision to make on your own.

Diet Creep: How Old Habits Return

This is probably the most common reason for weight regain

on medication. Diet creep is the gradual, often unconscious return to old eating patterns and portion sizes.

In the beginning, you were vigilant. You tracked everything. You measured portions. You were mindful about every food choice. But as time went on and the medication was working, you relaxed. You stopped tracking as carefully. You eyeballed portions instead of measuring. You added back foods you'd been avoiding. You started having treats more regularly.

Each individual change is small. A slightly larger portion of rice. An extra snack in the afternoon. A glass of wine most nights instead of occasionally. Weekend eating that's a bit more indulgent. None of it feels significant in the moment. But cumulatively, these small increases add up to several hundred extra calories per day. Over weeks and months, that causes weight regain.

Diet creep often happens so gradually that you don't notice it. You're not consciously deciding to eat more. You're just being a bit less strict, a bit less vigilant. The medication is still suppressing your appetite to some degree, so you're not feeling out of control. But you're eating more than you were during active weight loss.

This is especially common once you've hit your initial goal or gotten close to it. The urgency and motivation that drove you in the beginning has faded. You feel like you can relax a bit. And relaxing is fine for maintenance, but if you relax too much, regain happens.

The solution is to get honest with yourself about what you're actually eating. Go back to tracking for at least a week, maybe two. Measure portions again. Log everything. This will show you whether your intake has crept up from where it was during successful weight loss.

Often, people are shocked to discover they're eating 300 to 500 calories more per day than they thought. Those calories are the difference between maintaining and slowly regaining.

Once you have accurate data, you can make informed decisions about adjustments. You don't necessarily need to go back to the strictest version of your eating. But you do need to find a level of intake that maintains your weight rather than causing gradual regain.

Addressing the Underlying Behaviors

Weight regain isn't just about food and metabolism. It's often about behaviors and habits that drove weight gain in the first place resurfacing.

Maybe you're eating in response to stress again. Maybe you're using food for comfort when you're sad or bored. Maybe you're eating mindlessly in front of the TV. Maybe social eating has gotten out of hand. Whatever patterns contributed to weight gain before can come back, even with medication on board.

The medication suppresses physical hunger. It doesn't change the psychological or emotional drivers of eating. If you haven't addressed those underlying behaviors and patterns, they'll reassert themselves over time.

This is where the work of examining your relationship with food becomes important. Why do you eat when you're not hungry? What triggers overeating for you? What emotions or situations lead you to food? What purposes does food serve in your life beyond nutrition?

These are hard questions, and answering them honestly requires self-reflection and often professional help. A therapist who specializes in eating behaviors can help you identify patterns and develop healthier coping mechanisms that don't involve food.

Support groups, whether in-person or online, can also be valuable. Talking with others who are going through similar experiences can help you feel less alone and can provide practical strategies for dealing with challenges.

The point is, medication alone isn't a permanent solution if the underlying behaviors that caused weight gain in the first place aren't addressed. The medication gives you a window of opportunity to work on those behaviors without the constant burden of hunger. But the work still needs to happen.

When Switching Medications Might Help (Doctor's Decision)

If you've tightened up your eating, increased your activity, addressed lifestyle factors, and you're still regaining weight despite being on your GLP-1 medication, it might be time to talk to your doctor about options.

One option is increasing your dose if you're not already at the maximum. If you're on a lower or moderate dose and your appetite suppression has diminished, a higher dose might help. Your doctor can evaluate whether this is appropriate based on your response, side effects, and overall health.

Another option is switching to a different GLP-1 medication. Some people respond better to tirzepatide than semaglutide, or vice versa. If you've been on one for a long time and it seems less effective now, switching might produce a renewed response. This isn't guaranteed to work, but for some people it makes a difference.

Your doctor might also consider adding another medication to your regimen. Combining a GLP-1 with another weight loss medication can sometimes enhance results. This is more common in clinical weight loss practices than in general primary care, so you might need to see a specialist to explore this option.

It's also worth evaluating whether other medications you're taking might be interfering. If you started a new medication around the time weight regain began, that could be a factor. Your doctor might be able to switch you to an alternative that doesn't affect weight.

Before making any medication changes, your doctor will want to see evidence that you've been consistent with diet and exercise. They'll want to rule out other factors like thyroid issues or significant life changes that could explain the regain. Medication adjustments are usually considered after other strategies have been tried.

Never make medication changes on your own. Adjusting doses or switching medications without medical guidance can be dangerous and can create problems that are hard to fix. Always work with your healthcare provider on these decisions.

Taking Action Before Regain Becomes Significant

The best time to address weight regain is when it's small. If you've regained five pounds, that's much easier to reverse than if you've regained twenty or thirty pounds.

Weigh yourself regularly during maintenance. At least once a week, ideally at the same time under the same conditions. This isn't about obsessing over daily fluctuations. It's about catching an upward trend early.

Set a threshold for action. Decide in advance that if you regain a certain amount, maybe five pounds above your maintenance range, you'll immediately go back to stricter tracking and more intentional eating. Don't wait until regain is substantial to take action.

Be honest with yourself about what's changed. If you've regained weight, something has changed. Maybe it's your eating. Maybe it's your activity. Maybe it's stress or sleep or a medical issue. Figure out what it is and address it directly.

Don't panic and don't give up. Weight regain is frustrating, but it's not the end of the world. It doesn't mean you've failed or that all your progress is lost. It means you need to make some adjustments. That's completely doable.

Reach out for support when you need it. Talk to your doctor. Work with a dietitian or therapist. Connect with others who understand. You don't have to figure this out alone.

Weight regain while on medication can feel especially disheartening because the medication was supposed to make this easier. And it does make it easier. But it doesn't make it effortless, and it doesn't eliminate the need for ongoing attention to eating, movement, and lifestyle. The medication is a powerful tool, but it works best when you're actively using all the other tools at your disposal too.

In the next chapter, we'll look at special considerations for specific populations. People dealing with PCOS, menopause, older adults, athletes, and others who might need slightly different approaches to optimize their results on GLP-1 medications.

Chapter 13
For Specific Populations

GLP-1 medications work for a wide range of people, but not everyone's situation is identical. Age, medical conditions, activity level, and hormonal status all affect how you respond to these medications and what strategies work best for optimizing your results.

This chapter addresses specific populations who might need to approach things differently than the general guidelines we've covered so far.

Older Adults: Muscle Preservation Priorities

If you're over sixty, or even over fifty, losing weight on GLP-1 medications requires extra attention to muscle preservation. Age-related muscle loss, called sarcopenia, accelerates as we get older. Combine that with rapid weight loss, and you can lose muscle mass at an alarming rate if you're not careful.

Muscle matters more as you age. It's not just about appearance. Muscle mass is directly tied to your ability to stay independent, prevent falls, recover from illness or injury, and maintain quality of life. Older adults who lose significant muscle mass face increased risk of disability, frailty, and loss of independence.

The challenge is that older adults often need more protein than younger people to maintain muscle, but appetite tends to decrease with age even before adding a GLP-1 medication into the mix. When you combine natural age-related appetite reduction with medication-induced appetite suppression, getting adequate protein becomes really difficult.

Older adults should aim for the higher end of protein recommendations. Target at least 1.0 to 1.2 grams of protein per kilogram of body weight, and possibly higher if you're very active or losing weight rapidly. For a 150-pound person, that's roughly 68 to 82 grams minimum, but aiming for 90 to 110 grams would be better.

Resistance training is absolutely critical for older adults on GLP-1 medications. Not optional, not something to get to eventually. Critical. Lift weights, use resistance bands, do bodyweight exercises at least two to three times per week. This signals your body to preserve muscle even during weight loss.

If you're new to resistance training or have mobility limitations, work with a physical therapist or trainer who specializes in older adults. They can design a program that's safe and effective for your current fitness level and any physical limitations you have.

Slower weight loss is actually better for older adults. Losing weight very rapidly increases the likelihood of excessive muscle loss. If you can lose weight at a moderate pace of one to two pounds per week rather than three to four pounds, that's preferable for preserving muscle and bone density.

Bone health deserves attention too. Weight loss can affect bone density, especially in older adults who are already at higher risk for osteoporosis. Make sure you're getting adequate calcium and vitamin D. Weight-bearing exercise helps maintain bone density. Discuss bone density testing with your doctor if you're losing significant weight.

Be cautious about becoming too lean. While obesity carries health risks, being significantly underweight or having very low body fat also carries risks for older adults. Having some extra weight can actually be protective in older age. Don't chase an aggressive goal weight that might leave you too thin.

PCOS and Hormonal Considerations

Polycystic ovary syndrome creates unique challenges for weight loss because it involves both hormonal imbalances and insulin resistance. Women with PCOS often have elevated testosterone, irregular periods, insulin resistance, and difficulty losing weight even with significant effort.

The good news is that GLP-1 medications can be particularly effective for women with PCOS because they address the insulin resistance component. Improving insulin sensitivity helps with both weight loss and hormonal balance. Some women find that their periods become more regular and other PCOS symptoms improve as they lose weight on these medications.

However, weight loss might still be slower for women with PCOS compared to women without it. You might need to be more careful about carbohydrate intake since insulin resistance makes it harder to process carbohydrates efficiently. This doesn't necessarily mean going very low carb, but it does mean being mindful about carb quality and portions.

Pairing carbohydrates with protein and fat helps moderate blood sugar response. Choose complex carbohydrates like whole grains, legumes, and vegetables over refined carbs. Watch portions of even healthy carbs like fruit, rice, and potatoes.

Exercise is especially important for managing PCOS. Both resistance training and cardio help improve insulin sensitivity. Some research suggests that interval training might be particularly beneficial for women with PCOS.

If you're working with an endocrinologist or PCOS specialist, they might prescribe metformin alongside your GLP-1 medication. The combination can be effective for addressing insulin resistance and supporting weight loss.

Birth control pills or other hormone-regulating medications might also be part of your treatment plan. Discuss with your doctor how these medications interact with your GLP-1 medication and whether adjustments are needed.

Don't compare your progress to women without PCOS. Your timeline might be different, and that's okay. Focus on the fact that you're making progress, even if it's slower than you'd like.

Binge Eating Disorder: Different Strategies Needed

Binge eating disorder is characterized by episodes of eating large amounts of food in a short period, feeling out of control during these episodes, and experiencing distress afterward. It's the most common eating disorder, and it's different from occasional overeating or emotional eating.

GLP-1 medications can help reduce binge episodes for some people by reducing overall appetite and food preoccupation. The physical urge to binge can be less intense when appetite is suppressed. Some research suggests these medications might be particularly helpful for binge eating disorder.

However, medication alone isn't sufficient treatment for BED. The psychological and behavioral components need to be addressed too. Binge eating often has roots in emotional regulation, trauma, restriction patterns, or other psychological factors. Medication doesn't resolve those underlying issues.

If you have binge eating disorder and you're taking a GLP-1 medication, you should also be working with a therapist who specializes in eating disorders. Cognitive behavioral therapy has strong evidence for treating BED. Dialectical behavior therapy can also be effective, particularly if emotion regulation is a major factor.

Be careful about restriction. Ironically, being too restrictive with food, even unintentionally because of appetite suppression, can trigger binge episodes. Your body and brain might interpret severe restriction as a threat, leading to compensatory binge eating when the medication's effects wear off temporarily or when you're in a triggering situation.

Make sure you're eating enough even when you're not hungry. If you're consistently eating very little because the medication kills your appetite, this can set up a restrict-binge cycle. Aim for regular meals with adequate calories and nutrition even if you have to eat mechanically without hunger driving you.

Work on identifying binge triggers and developing coping strategies that don't involve food. If stress triggers binges, find stress management techniques. If certain situations or emotions trigger binges, work with your therapist on strategies for managing those situations differently.

Don't rely solely on the medication to prevent binges. Use it as a tool to make recovery easier, but continue doing the therapeutic work necessary for long-term management of BED.

Diabetics: Balancing Blood Sugar and Weight Goals

If you have type 2 diabetes, you might be taking a GLP-1

medication primarily for blood sugar control rather than weight loss. But weight loss is often a welcome bonus since losing weight improves insulin sensitivity and blood sugar control.

The challenge for diabetics is balancing weight loss goals with blood sugar management. Losing weight too quickly can affect blood sugar levels unpredictably. If you're on other diabetes medications, particularly insulin or sulfonylureas, rapid weight loss and reduced food intake can cause low blood sugar episodes.

Monitor your blood sugar closely, especially in the first few months of starting a GLP-1 medication or when increasing the dose. Check your levels more frequently than usual. Watch for symptoms of hypoglycemia like shakiness, sweating, confusion, or dizziness.

Your other diabetes medications might need adjustment as you lose weight. As your insulin sensitivity improves, you might need less insulin or lower doses of other medications. Work closely with your doctor on medication adjustments. Don't make changes on your own.

Be strategic about carbohydrate intake. You don't need to eliminate carbs, but managing portions and choosing complex carbs over simple ones helps keep blood sugar more stable. Pairing carbs with protein and healthy fats slows digestion and prevents blood sugar spikes.

If you're having low blood sugar episodes, you need to

treat them appropriately even though it might feel like it's interfering with weight loss. Keep fast-acting carbs available like glucose tablets or juice. Treat lows when they happen. Your safety is more important than the scale.

Don't let weight loss goals cause you to under-eat to the point where blood sugar becomes dangerously unstable. Adequate, regular meals help keep blood sugar more predictable. Skipping meals or eating very little might seem like it would help with weight loss, but it can create blood sugar swings that are dangerous for diabetics.

Celebrate improvements in blood sugar control and A1C even if weight loss is slower than you'd like. Better blood sugar control is the primary goal. Weight loss is a beneficial side effect that supports that goal.

Post-Menopausal Women: Unique Challenges

Menopause changes how your body processes food, stores fat, and responds to weight loss efforts. Declining estrogen affects metabolism, appetite regulation, where fat is stored, and how easily you lose weight.

After menopause, many women find that weight loss becomes harder and that fat shifts to the abdominal area rather than hips and thighs. This visceral fat around organs is particularly concerning from a health standpoint because it's associated with increased risk of heart disease and diabetes.

GLP-1 medications can definitely work for post-menopausal

women, but weight loss might be slower than for younger women. Your metabolism is naturally slower after menopause. You might need to be more patient and accept a more gradual rate of loss.

Strength training becomes even more important after menopause. Declining estrogen accelerates muscle loss. Maintaining muscle through resistance training helps preserve metabolism, bone density, and functional strength. Aim for at least two to three sessions per week.

Bone health requires attention. Menopause increases risk of osteoporosis, and weight loss can potentially accelerate bone loss if you're not careful. Make sure you're getting adequate calcium and vitamin D. Include weight-bearing exercise. Discuss bone density testing with your doctor.

Sleep disturbances are common after menopause, with hot flashes and night sweats disrupting sleep. Poor sleep affects hunger hormones and makes weight loss harder. Address sleep issues proactively. Keep your bedroom cool. Use moisture-wicking sleepwear. Consider discussing hormone replacement therapy with your doctor if sleep disturbances are severe.

Some post-menopausal women benefit from hormone replacement therapy, which can help with weight management, sleep, mood, and other menopausal symptoms. This is a complex decision with potential benefits and risks. Discuss thoroughly with your doctor whether it might be appropriate for you.

Be realistic about body composition changes. Your body at sixty doesn't have the same ability to achieve or maintain very low body fat as it did at thirty. That's normal and okay. Focus on being healthy and strong rather than chasing an unrealistic aesthetic standard.

Athletes and Active Individuals

If you're very physically active or training for athletic performance, using GLP-1 medications for weight loss requires careful consideration. The appetite suppression that helps others can work against you if it prevents you from eating enough to fuel your training.

Athletes need adequate calories and nutrients to support training, recovery, and performance. Under-eating can lead to overtraining syndrome, increased injury risk, hormonal disruptions, and decreased performance. The challenge is balancing weight loss goals with athletic performance goals.

If you're an athlete considering a GLP-1 medication, be clear about your priorities. Are you trying to lose weight for health reasons? For performance in a weight-class sport? For aesthetics? Understanding your primary goal helps determine whether using these medications makes sense.

For athletes who do use GLP-1 medications, careful attention to nutrition timing is critical. You might need to eat on a schedule rather than relying on hunger cues, since the medication suppresses appetite even when your body genuinely needs fuel.

Time your meals around training. Make sure you're eating adequate carbohydrates before intense workouts for energy and after workouts for recovery. Protein timing matters too. Get protein within a few hours after resistance training.

Your protein needs are higher than sedentary individuals. Active people need at least 1.6 to 2.2 grams of protein per kilogram of body weight, possibly more during weight loss. For a 150-pound athlete, that's roughly 109 to 150 grams per day.

Monitor performance markers. If your strength is declining, your endurance is suffering, your recovery is poor, or you're getting injured more frequently, you're probably not eating enough. Adjust your intake upward even if it slows weight loss.

Consider whether you actually need to lose weight. Many athletes are already at healthy weights and body compositions. Using weight loss medication to achieve extremely low body fat might compromise health and performance. Discuss with a sports nutritionist or sports medicine doctor whether weight loss is actually beneficial for you.

If you're losing weight to make a weight class for competition, work with professionals who understand the specific demands of your sport. Don't use GLP-1 medications as a shortcut for rapid weight cuts, as this can be dangerous.

Some athletes use these medications during off-seasons to lose fat while maintaining training at a lower intensity, then discontinue during competitive seasons when maximal performance is required. This requires medical supervision and careful planning.

General Considerations Across Populations

Regardless of which population you fall into, some principles apply universally when using GLP-1 medications.

Work with healthcare providers who understand your specific situation. If you have PCOS, see an endocrinologist who specializes in hormonal disorders. If you're an older adult, make sure your doctor considers age-related factors. If you have diabetes, your diabetes management should be the priority.

Don't assume that general guidelines apply perfectly to you. You might need modifications based on your age, health conditions, activity level, or other factors. Be willing to experiment and adjust based on how your body responds.

Monitor your progress with measures beyond just the scale. Health markers, body composition, strength, energy levels, and how you feel all matter. Don't let scale weight be the only measure of success.

Be patient. If you're in one of these populations, your progress might be slower than the averages cited in studies. That doesn't mean the medication isn't working or that you're doing something wrong. It just means your situation is more complex.

Advocate for yourself. If something doesn't feel right, if your progress has stalled, if you're experiencing concerning symptoms, speak up. You know your body better than anyone else. Trust your instincts and push for answers when needed.

In the next section of the book, we'll pull everything together with practical protocols you can follow and strategies for long-term success. We'll give you actionable steps to take regardless of your specific situation.

PART 5

Putting It All Together

Chapter 14
Your 30-Day Optimization Protocol

You've read through thirteen chapters of information, strategies, and troubleshooting advice. Now it's time to put it all into action. This chapter gives you a structured 30-day protocol to optimize your results on GLP-1 medications.

This protocol works whether you're just starting your medication, you've been on it for months and want to restart with better habits, or you've hit a plateau and need to get things back on track. It's designed to be manageable, focusing on one key area each week so you don't get overwhelmed trying to change everything at once.

Week 1: Assessment and Baseline

The first week is about gathering information. You can't improve what you don't measure, and you can't know what to fix if you don't understand your starting point.

Day 1-2: Body Metrics

Weigh yourself first thing in the morning after using the bathroom. Record this number. If you have access to a body composition scale or can get a body composition assessment, do that too. It's helpful to know your starting body fat percentage and lean mass.

Take measurements with a tape measure. Record your waist at the narrowest point, hips at the widest point, thighs mid-way up, and upper arms. These numbers will show progress even when the scale doesn't move.

Take progress photos. Front, side, and back views in form-fitting clothes or workout attire. Yes, this feels uncomfortable. Do it anyway. Photos reveal changes that you can't see in the mirror because you look at yourself every day.

Day 3-7: Food Tracking

Track everything you eat and drink for the entire week. Don't change your eating habits yet. Just observe and record. Use an app like MyFitnessPal, Cronometer, or Lose It. Measure and weigh food when possible for accuracy, but at minimum, make honest estimates.

This baseline tracking shows you how much you're actually eating, where your calories are coming from, how much protein you're getting, and what patterns exist in your eating. You might be surprised by what you discover.

At the end of the week, review your food logs and calculate

your daily averages for total calories, protein, carbs, and fat. Look for patterns. Do you eat differently on weekends? Are you getting enough protein? Are there times of day when you consistently overeat? Are there trigger foods that lead to eating more than intended?

Day 1-7: Activity Baseline

Track your daily steps using your phone or a fitness tracker. Note any formal exercise you do. Get a baseline for how much you're currently moving. Don't change anything yet, just observe.

If you have a fitness tracker that measures heart rate or active minutes, pay attention to that data too. It gives you a fuller picture of your activity level.

Day 1-7: Lifestyle Assessment

Keep a simple log of your sleep. What time you went to bed, what time you woke up, approximately how many hours you slept. Rate your sleep quality on a scale of 1 to 10.

Note your stress levels each day on a scale of 1 to 10. Notice what situations or factors increase stress.

Track alcohol consumption if applicable. How many drinks per week? On what days?

Notice energy levels throughout the day. Do you have consistent energy or are there crashes? When do you feel best and worst?

Week 1 Wrap-Up

At the end of week one, you should have a clear picture of your current situation. You know your measurements and weight. You know what and how much you're eating. You know your activity level. You have data on sleep, stress, and other lifestyle factors.

This is your baseline. Everything moving forward will be measured against this starting point.

Week 2: Protein and Tracking Focus

Week two is all about optimizing your protein intake and tightening up your food tracking. These are the two foundational nutritional habits that have the biggest impact on your results.

Setting Your Protein Target

Based on your current weight and goals, calculate your protein target. Aim for 0.7 to 1.0 grams of protein per pound of your goal body weight. If you currently weigh 180 pounds and your goal weight is 150 pounds, your target is roughly 105 to 150 grams per day. Start with the lower end if that feels more manageable, knowing you can increase it later.

Day 8-14: Hit Your Protein Target Daily

Every single day this week, your goal is to hit your protein target. Plan your meals around protein sources. Eat protein first at every meal before anything else.

Stock your kitchen with high-protein foods. Chicken breast, fish, lean beef, eggs, Greek yogurt, cottage cheese, protein powder, and other lean protein sources. Make sure you always have easy protein options available.

Use protein shakes strategically if needed. If you're struggling to get enough protein from food alone, have a protein shake once or twice a day. This makes hitting your target much easier.

Spread protein throughout the day. Aim for 25 to 40 grams at each meal rather than trying to get all your protein in one or two meals. Your body uses protein more effectively when it's distributed across multiple eating occasions.

Continuing Food Tracking

Keep tracking everything you eat, just like you did in week one. But now you're not just observing. You're actively trying to hit specific targets. Stay at or slightly below the calorie level you averaged in week one if you're trying to lose weight. Focus primarily on hitting protein, then let carbs and fat fall where they may within your calorie budget.

Week 2 Wrap-Up

By the end of week two, hitting your protein target should start feeling more natural. You've figured out which foods work best for you. You've established a pattern of planning meals around protein. And you're tracking consistently, which creates accountability and awareness.

Week 3: Movement and NEAT

Week three adds movement to the equation. You're going to increase both your formal exercise and your daily activity level.

Day 15-21: Resistance Training

If you're not already doing resistance training, start this week with two sessions. Schedule them in advance. Monday and Thursday, or Tuesday and Friday, whatever works for your schedule. Put them on your calendar as non-negotiable appointments.

If you've never done resistance training before, start simple. Bodyweight exercises like squats, push-ups, lunges, and planks are fine. You can find beginner routines on YouTube or use an app like Nike Training Club or Fitbod.

If you have gym access, use machines or free weights. Focus on compound movements that work multiple muscle groups: squats, deadlifts, bench press, rows, shoulder press. Three sets of 8 to 12 reps for each exercise is a good starting point.

Each session should last 30 to 45 minutes. You don't need to spend hours in the gym. Quality over quantity.

If you're already doing resistance training, continue your current routine or increase intensity slightly. Maybe add a third session this week or increase the weight you're lifting.

Day 15-21: Increasing NEAT

Set a daily step goal that's higher than your week-one baseline. If you averaged 4,000 steps per day in week one, aim for 6,000 steps per day this week. If you averaged 7,000, aim for 9,000.

Find ways to add movement throughout your day. Take a 10-minute walk after each meal. Walk while talking on the phone. Take the stairs instead of the elevator. Park farther away. Set a timer to get up and move for five minutes every hour if you have a desk job.

Track your steps daily. Celebrate when you hit your goal. If you miss your goal one day, don't beat yourself up. Just get back on track the next day.

Optional: Add Cardio

If you enjoy cardio and you have time, add one or two cardio sessions this week. Walking, cycling, swimming, hiking, whatever you enjoy. Aim for 20 to 40 minutes per session. This is optional, not required. Resistance training and daily steps are the priorities.

Week 3 Wrap-Up

By the end of week three, you should have established an exercise routine. You've done at least two resistance training sessions and increased your daily movement. Your body is adapting to this new activity level. You might feel sore, especially if you're new to resistance training. That's normal. Keep moving, stay hydrated, and prioritize protein for recovery.

Week 4: Fine-Tuning and Troubleshooting

Week four is about adjusting based on what you've learned in the previous three weeks. You're going to review your progress, identify what's working and what's not, and make strategic tweaks.

Day 22: Progress Assessment

Weigh yourself under the same conditions as day one. Take measurements again. Take new progress photos. Compare everything to your baseline from week one.

Calculate your averages for week three. How many calories per day? How much protein? How many steps? How many workouts?

Evaluate how you feel. Energy levels, mood, hunger, satiety, strength, sleep quality. Has anything improved compared to week one?

Day 23-28: Adjust and Optimize

Based on your week-four assessment, make adjustments.

If you lost weight and feel good, keep doing what you're

doing. If weight loss was slower than expected, consider reducing calories slightly or increasing activity. If you're losing weight too fast or feeling exhausted, increase calories slightly.

If you struggled to hit your protein target, troubleshoot why. Do you need more protein shakes? Different protein sources? Better meal planning?

If you didn't hit your step goal consistently, identify barriers. Do you need to wake up earlier to fit in a morning walk? Do you need reminders to move throughout the day?

If you skipped workouts, figure out why. Was the time of day wrong? Was the workout too long or too hard? Do you need a different type of exercise?

Make one or two specific changes based on your assessment. Don't try to fix everything at once. Pick the biggest issue and address that.

Day 22-28: Address Lifestyle Factors

If sleep was poor during weeks one through three, prioritize improving it this week. Go to bed 30 minutes earlier. Create a better bedtime routine. Make your bedroom more conducive to sleep.

If stress was high, implement at least one stress-management technique this week. Morning meditation, evening walks, talking to a friend, whatever helps you decompress.

If alcohol has been an issue, reduce consumption this week. If you were having five drinks per week, cut it to two or three.

Notice how this affects your energy, sleep, and weight.

Creating Your Personalized Action Plan

By the end of the 30 days, you should have a clear action plan moving forward. Here's how to create it.

Identify Your Non-Negotiables

Based on the last 30 days, what habits made the biggest difference for you? What felt sustainable? These become your non-negotiables going forward. For most people, this includes daily protein targets, resistance training two to three times per week, and a daily step goal.

Set Specific Goals

Be specific about what you'll do, not just what you hope will happen. Instead of "lose weight," your goals might be "eat 120 grams of protein daily," "lift weights three times per week," "walk 8,000 steps daily," and "sleep 7.5 hours per night."

Plan for Obstacles

Identify potential obstacles to maintaining your habits and plan solutions in advance. Traveling for work? Pack protein shakes and resistance bands. Busy week coming up? Meal prep on Sunday. Social events scheduled? Decide in advance how you'll handle them.

Schedule Regular Check-Ins

Commit to weighing yourself weekly, tracking food at least a few days per week to stay accountable, and reassessing your plan monthly. Regular check-ins help you catch problems early before they derail your progress.

Build in Flexibility

Your plan should be sustainable long-term, which means it needs to accommodate real life. You'll have weeks where you can't hit every goal. That's okay. The plan should be your guide, not a rigid set of rules that creates stress and guilt when you can't follow them perfectly.

Troubleshooting Flowchart

Use this flowchart when you're stuck or not seeing the results you want.

Problem: Not losing weight or weight loss has stalled

Are you tracking food accurately?

☐ No → Start tracking everything for at least one week

☐ Yes → Continue to next question

Are you hitting your protein target most days?

☐ No → Focus on increasing protein for two weeks, then reassess

☐ Yes → Continue to next question

Are you in a calorie deficit?

☐ Not sure → Track carefully for one week and calculate your average intake vs. your estimated needs

☐ No → Reduce calories by 200-300 per day or increase activity

☐ Yes → Continue to next question

Are you doing resistance training at least twice per week?

☐ No → Start resistance training immediately

☐ Yes → Continue to next question

Are you getting adequate sleep (7+ hours)?

☐ No → Make sleep a priority for two weeks, then reassess

☐ Yes → Continue to next question

Are you managing stress reasonably well?

☐ No → Implement stress-management strategies

☐ Yes → Continue to next question

Could there be a metabolic or medical issue?

☐ Possible → Talk to your doctor about comprehensive testing

☐ Already ruled out → Consider that your current weight might be appropriate for your body, focus on body composition rather than scale weight

Problem: Constantly hungry despite medication

Are you on a therapeutic dose?

☐ No → Discuss dose increase with your doctor

☐ Yes → Continue to next question

Are you getting enough protein?

☐ No → Increase protein significantly for two weeks

☐ Yes → Continue to next question

Are you eating enough overall?

☐ No → Slightly increase calories, especially from protein and healthy fats

☐ Yes → Continue to next question

Are you sleeping enough?

☐ No → Improve sleep, as poor sleep increases hunger

☐ Yes → Continue to next question

Is hunger worse at specific times?

☐ Yes → Adjust meal timing to address those specific times

☐ No → Discuss with your doctor whether the medication is working properly for you

Problem: Feeling exhausted and weak

Are you eating enough overall?

☐ No → Increase calories, especially before/after workouts

☐ Yes → Continue to next question

Are you getting enough protein?
☐ No → Increase protein intake
☐ Yes → Continue to next question

Are you sleeping adequately?
☐ No → Prioritize sleep immediately
☐ Yes → Continue to next question

Have you had bloodwork recently?
☐ No → Ask your doctor to check thyroid, iron, vitamin D, and B12
☐ Yes, and it's normal → Consider reducing exercise intensity or frequency temporarily

Problem: Losing weight but not happy with body composition
Are you doing resistance training?
☐ No → Start immediately, this is essential
☐ Yes → Continue to next question

Are you getting enough protein?
☐ No → Increase protein to at least 1.0g per pound of goal weight
☐ Yes → Continue to next question

Have you been doing resistance training consistently for at least 8 weeks?

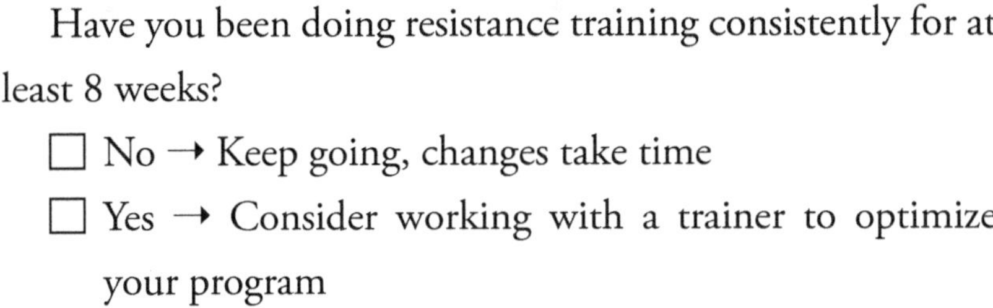

This 30-day protocol and troubleshooting approach give you a concrete path forward. You're not guessing about what to do next. You're following a systematic process that addresses the most important factors in order of priority.

The key to success is consistency, not perfection. You won't execute perfectly every day. That's expected. What matters is getting back on track quickly when you slip and maintaining the habits that matter most over time.

In the next chapter, we'll talk about strategies for long-term success beyond these first 30 days. How to maintain your habits, how to handle setbacks, and how to build a sustainable relationship with food and your body that lasts years, not just months.

Chapter 15
Long-Term Success Strategies

The first few months on a GLP-1 medication often feel relatively easy. The appetite suppression is strong. The weight comes off. Motivation is high. But real success isn't measured in the first three or six months. It's measured in years. Can you maintain your results? Can you sustain healthy habits? Can you build a life that feels good and supports your health long-term?

This chapter is about thinking beyond the initial weight loss phase and creating strategies that work for the long haul.

Building Habits That Outlast the Medication

Whether you stay on GLP-1 medications indefinitely or eventually transition off them, you need habits that don't depend entirely on appetite suppression to work.

The medication gives you a window of opportunity. While your appetite is suppressed, you have the mental and physical space to build new patterns around food, movement, and self-care. But if you rely completely on the medication to do all the work, you won't have developed the skills and habits needed to maintain your results if you ever stop taking it.

Think of the medication as training wheels. Training wheels make learning to ride a bike much easier. They prevent falls and build confidence. But eventually, the goal is to ride without them. Even if you end up keeping the training wheels on indefinitely, you're better off knowing how to balance on your own.

Start building habits now that could work even without medication. Plan and prepare meals in advance instead of relying on not being hungry to avoid overeating. Practice portion awareness by actually measuring food sometimes, not just eating small portions because you're too full to eat more. Develop a consistent exercise routine driven by schedule and commitment, not just by how you feel that day.

Create environmental supports that make healthy choices easier. Keep nutritious food readily available. Remove or limit access to foods that trigger overeating. Set up your home and workspace to encourage movement. These environmental factors continue supporting you regardless of medication status.

Build skills around emotional regulation that don't involve food. Learn to sit with uncomfortable emotions rather than eating to suppress them. Develop a toolkit of coping strategies for stress, boredom, sadness, and anxiety. The medication reduces physical hunger, but it doesn't teach you how to handle emotions without food. That's work you need to do separately.

Practice mindful eating even when you're not hungry. Pay attention to food. Eat without distraction sometimes. Notice flavors, textures, and satisfaction. These practices help you maintain a healthier relationship with food that persists beyond medication.

The goal is to reach a point where the medication is helpful but not absolutely essential. Where you've developed habits and skills that support maintaining your weight and health with or without it.

Maintenance Planning

Maintenance is harder than weight loss for a lot of people. During weight loss, you have clear goals and visible progress. Maintenance lacks that forward momentum. The scale isn't moving. You're just trying to stay where you are. It can feel less motivating.

But maintenance is where the real work happens. Anyone can lose weight for a few months with enough motivation and restriction. Maintaining that loss for years requires a completely different skill set.

Define what maintenance means for you. Is it staying within a five-pound range of your goal weight? Maintaining certain measurements? Fitting into specific clothes? Maintaining strength and fitness levels? Be specific about what you're maintaining.

Set maintenance goals that aren't just about weight. Focus on behaviors rather than outcomes. Your maintenance goals might include continuing to exercise three times per week, eating protein at every meal, getting adequate sleep, and tracking food a few days per week. These behavioral goals give you something concrete to work toward even when the scale isn't changing.

Create a maintenance calorie range. You figured out what calorie level causes weight loss for you. Maintenance will be higher than that, but probably not as high as what you were eating before you started losing weight. Find the calorie range that keeps your weight stable. This might take some experimentation.

Plan for inevitable fluctuations. Your weight will go up and down within a range. That's normal. Decide in advance what fluctuation range is acceptable and what will trigger action. If you maintain at 160 pounds, maybe anything between 158 and 163 is fine. But if you hit 165, that's your signal to tighten things up for a couple of weeks.

Keep tracking something. You don't need to track food every day forever, but tracking something keeps you accountable. Maybe you track food a few days per week. Maybe you track exercise and steps. Maybe you just weigh yourself weekly. Some form of monitoring helps catch problems before they become significant.

Stay connected to your why. Why did you want to lose weight in the first place? Health? Energy? Longevity? Feeling better in your body? Keep that motivation visible. Write it down. Revisit it regularly. When maintenance feels tedious, reconnecting with your why can renew your commitment.

Community and Support Systems

Long-term success is much easier with support. Very few people maintain significant weight loss completely alone. Having people who understand what you're going through makes a huge difference.

Find a community of people on similar journeys. This might be an online group for people taking GLP-1 medications. It might be a weight loss support group. It might be a fitness community. Somewhere you can share struggles, celebrate victories, and get encouragement when things are hard.

Online communities can be valuable because they're accessible anytime and often include people dealing with the exact same medication experiences. Reddit, Facebook groups, and forums dedicated to GLP-1 medications have thousands of members sharing experiences and advice.

But be selective about which communities you engage with. Some online spaces can be toxic, promoting unhealthy behaviors or creating unrealistic expectations. Look for communities that are supportive, evidence-based, and focused on sustainable health rather than extreme restriction or rapid weight loss at any cost.

In-person support can be powerful too. Weight Watchers, TOPS, Overeaters Anonymous, or local support groups through hospitals or clinics provide face-to-face connection. Some people find in-person accountability more meaningful than online interaction.

Build support within your existing relationships. Talk to friends and family about your journey. Let them know how they can support you. Be specific. Maybe support means not commenting on what you eat. Maybe it means joining you for walks. Maybe it means not keeping certain foods in the house. People who care about you want to help, but they might not know how unless you tell them.

Consider working with professionals as part of your support system. A registered dietitian, a therapist who specializes in eating and body image, or a personal trainer can provide expertise and accountability that friends and family can't offer.

Find an accountability partner. Someone who's also working on health goals. Check in with each other regularly. Share your challenges and progress. Having someone who's counting on you shows up creates extra motivation to follow through on commitments.

When to Seek Professional Help

Sometimes you need more support than you can get

from communities, friends, or self-help strategies. Knowing when to seek professional help can prevent small issues from becoming major problems.

Consider seeing a registered dietitian if you're struggling to meet nutritional needs on reduced food intake, if you have complex dietary requirements due to medical conditions, if you need help planning meals or figuring out portions, or if you're confused about what to eat.

A dietitian who specializes in weight management and GLP-1 medications can be particularly helpful. They understand the unique challenges these medications create and can provide practical strategies tailored to your situation.

Consider seeing a therapist if emotional eating is a significant issue, if you're dealing with body image struggles, if weight loss is bringing up unexpected emotions or past trauma, if you have a history of disordered eating, if you're using food to cope with stress, anxiety, or depression, or if your relationship with food feels obsessive or out of control.

Therapy isn't just for people with diagnosed mental health conditions. It's for anyone who wants support working through challenges. A therapist specializing in eating behaviors, body image, or health behavior change can help you develop healthier patterns.

Consider seeing an endocrinologist or obesity medicine specialist if you're not responding to the medication as expected, if you have complex metabolic issues like thyroid problems or PCOS, if you're on multiple medications and need coordination of care, or if your primary care doctor isn't sure how to optimize your treatment.

Consider working with a personal trainer if you're new to exercise and need guidance on proper form and program design, if you've plateaued and need help intensifying your workouts, if you have injuries or limitations that require modified exercises, or if you need accountability to show up consistently.

Don't wait until things are desperate to seek help. Early intervention is easier and more effective than trying to fix major problems after they've been going on for months or years.

Many people hesitate to seek professional help because of cost. But consider the cost of not getting help. If struggling alone leads to regaining all your weight, developing health complications, or years of frustration, that costs far more than a few sessions with a professional.

Check whether your insurance covers dietitian visits, therapy, or medical weight management. Many plans do, especially if you have diabetes or other obesity-related conditions. If insurance doesn't cover it, ask about sliding scale fees or payment plans.

Measuring Success Beyond the Scale

The scale is useful data, but it's not the only measure

of success. In fact, over-reliance on scale weight can be demoralizing and might cause you to miss other important indicators of progress and health.

Health markers matter more than weight. Blood pressure, blood sugar, cholesterol, inflammatory markers. These numbers directly reflect your health risk. Someone at a slightly higher weight with excellent health markers is healthier than someone at a lower weight with poor metabolic health.

Track your health markers regularly. Get bloodwork done at least annually. Celebrate improvements even if the scale isn't moving as fast as you'd like. Reducing your A1C, getting off blood pressure medication, or improving your cholesterol profile are huge wins.

How you feel is a valid measure of success. Do you have more energy? Better sleep? Less joint pain? Improved mood? Can you do activities you couldn't do before? These quality of life improvements matter tremendously.

Strength and fitness are important metrics. Can you lift heavier weights than you could three months ago? Can you walk farther without getting tired? Can you do more push-ups or hold a plank longer? These improvements show that you're getting healthier and stronger even if weight isn't changing.

Body composition tells a better story than weight alone. If you're losing fat and gaining muscle, you might not lose much weight, but you're transforming your body. Measurements, progress photos, and how clothes fit reveal these changes better than the scale.

Non-scale victories deserve celebration. Wearing clothes you haven't fit into in years. Walking up stairs without getting winded. Playing with your kids or grandkids without exhaustion. Sitting comfortably in an airplane seat. Feeling confident in photos. These victories are real and meaningful.

Keep a list of non-scale victories. Write them down when they happen. Refer back to this list when you're feeling discouraged about the number on the scale. It reminds you that success is much bigger than one metric.

Creating a Sustainable Relationship With Food

One of the most important aspects of long-term success is developing a relationship with food that's healthy, balanced, and sustainable. This means moving away from all-or-nothing thinking and finding a middle ground that works for your life.

Food is not the enemy. You need food to live. It provides energy, nutrients, pleasure, and social connection. The goal isn't to fear food or view it as something to be controlled and restricted at all times. The goal is to have a peaceful, functional relationship with food where you can enjoy it without it controlling you.

Reject diet mentality. You're not on a diet. Diets have start dates and end dates. They involve rules, restriction, and usually failure. You're making sustainable lifestyle changes. Some of those changes involve being thoughtful about food choices and portions, but it's not temporary restriction. It's finding a way of eating that you can maintain indefinitely.

Allow all foods in moderation. Labeling foods as "good" or "bad," "allowed" or "forbidden" sets up deprivation that often leads to bingeing. Instead, all foods can fit in a healthy eating pattern. Some foods you'll eat frequently because they're nutritious and support your goals. Other foods you'll eat occasionally because you enjoy them. But nothing is completely off limits.

Practice flexible eating. Some days you'll eat perfectly on plan. Other days you'll eat more or differently than planned. Both are okay. One meal or one day doesn't define your success. It's the overall pattern over weeks and months that matters.

Learn to eat for satisfaction, not just fullness or restriction. On GLP-1 medications, you might not feel traditionally hungry or full. But you can still notice what foods satisfy you, what tastes good, what makes you feel energized. Pay attention to satisfaction rather than just stopping when you're not hungry or eating just because it's mealtime.

Make peace with hunger. If you eventually reduce or stop your medication, hunger will return. This is normal and not something to fear. Hunger is just your body's signal that it needs energy. You can feel hunger without immediately needing to eat. You can tolerate some hunger between meals without it being an emergency.

Similarly, make peace with fullness. It's okay to feel comfortably full after a meal. You don't need to eat until you're stuffed, but you also don't need to be afraid of fullness. Find the level of satisfaction that feels good for your body.

Stop eating when you've had enough, not when you've finished everything on your plate. It's okay to leave food. It's okay to save leftovers. You don't need to force yourself to eat food just because it's there.

Give yourself permission to enjoy food. Eating isn't just about nutrition. It's also about pleasure, culture, celebration, and connection. Don't feel guilty for enjoying delicious food. Savor it. Appreciate it. Then move on with your day.

Mental Health Considerations

Your mental health affects your ability to maintain healthy habits, and your weight loss journey affects your mental health. These things are deeply interconnected.

Weight loss can improve mental health for many people. Feeling better physically, accomplishing a challenging goal, and improving health markers often boost mood and self-esteem. But weight loss can also bring up difficult emotions or create new challenges.

Some people experience anxiety about maintaining their weight loss. They fear regaining weight. They become hypervigilant about food and weight. This anxiety can interfere with quality of life and ironically might make maintenance harder because it's not sustainable to live in constant fear.

Body image issues don't automatically resolve with weight loss. You might have expected to feel completely different in your new body, but many people find that their negative self-perception persists even after significant weight loss. This can be disappointing and confusing.

If you've used food to cope with emotions for a long time, losing that coping mechanism can be difficult. The medication reduces physical hunger, but it doesn't fix the emotional reasons you were eating. You might find yourself struggling with emotions you were previously numbing with food.

Identity shifts can be challenging. If being overweight was part of how you saw yourself for a long time, changing your body changes your identity. This can feel disorienting. You might grieve aspects of your old self even while being happy about your progress.

Relationships can become complicated. Some partners feel threatened by your weight loss. Friends who also struggle with weight might distance themselves. You might receive unwanted attention or comments about your body. Navigating these relationship changes requires emotional energy.

All of these mental health considerations are normal. You're not broken or doing something wrong if weight loss brings up complex emotions. It's a major life change, and major changes come with psychological adjustment.

Take your mental health seriously. If you're struggling with anxiety, depression, disordered eating thoughts, or body image issues, get help. Don't assume these issues will resolve on their own or that you should just be able to power through them.

Practice self-compassion. You're doing something difficult. You'll have setbacks. You'll make mistakes. You'll have days where everything feels hard. That's part of being human. Treat yourself with the same kindness and understanding you'd offer a good friend going through the same thing.

Celebrate your progress without making your worth dependent on it. You're a valuable person regardless of your weight, your eating habits, or your exercise consistency. Your worth is inherent, not earned through achievement or self-improvement.

Creating Your Long-Term Vision

Think beyond the next few months. What does long-term success look like for you? Not just a number on the scale, but a life that feels good and sustainable.

Imagine yourself five years from now having successfully maintained your health improvements. What habits are you consistently doing? How do you handle challenging situations? What has become easy that used to be hard? What support systems are in place?

Write this vision down. Be specific. The clearer your vision of long-term success, the easier it is to make decisions today that align with that future.

Then work backward. What needs to happen in the next year to move you toward that five-year vision? What needs to happen in the next month? What needs to happen today?

This isn't about perfection or having everything figured out. It's about having a direction. A sense of where you're headed. The specific path will adjust as you go. But knowing generally where you want to end up helps you navigate the challenges along the way.

Long-term success is absolutely possible. Thousands of people maintain significant weight loss for years or decades. You can be one of them. It requires ongoing attention, consistent habits, support, and self-compassion. But it's doable. And it's worth it.

In the final chapter, we'll give you questions to ask your healthcare provider to make sure you're getting the support and monitoring you need for safe, effective long-term use of GLP-1 medications.

Chapter 16
Questions to Ask Your Healthcare Provider

Your relationship with your healthcare provider is crucial to your success on GLP-1 medications. These are powerful drugs that require medical supervision, monitoring, and ongoing communication. Being an informed, proactive patient helps ensure you get the care you need.

This chapter gives you the tools to have productive conversations with your doctor and know when to ask questions or raise concerns.

How to Be an Informed Patient

Being an informed patient doesn't mean self-diagnosing or second-guessing your doctor on everything. It means coming to appointments prepared, asking thoughtful questions, being honest about your experiences, and actively participating in your care.

Before appointments, write down what you want to discuss.

When you're sitting in the exam room, it's easy to forget what you wanted to ask. A written list ensures you cover everything important.

Bring data to appointments. If you've been tracking food, weight, exercise, or side effects, bring that information. Concrete data gives your doctor much better information than general statements like "I'm not losing much weight."

Be completely honest about adherence. If you've been skipping doses, drinking alcohol regularly, not exercising, or struggling with any aspect of the plan, tell your doctor. They can't help you if they don't know what's really happening. There's no judgment in acknowledging challenges.

Ask for clarification if you don't understand something. Medical terminology can be confusing. If your doctor says something you don't fully grasp, say "Can you explain that in a different way?" or "I want to make sure I understand. Are you saying..." A good doctor will appreciate your effort to understand and will take time to explain.

Take notes during appointments or ask if you can record the conversation. You'll forget some of what's discussed, especially if you're anxious or if a lot of information is covered. Notes help you remember instructions and recommendations.

Don't leave appointments with unanswered questions. If something is still unclear when the appointment is wrapping up, speak up. It's better to take an extra few minutes now than to spend weeks confused or worried.

Questions to Ask When Starting a GLP-1 Medication

If you're just beginning treatment, these questions help you understand what to expect and how to use the medication safely.

"What dose am I starting with, and how will we titrate up?" Understanding the titration schedule helps you know when to expect dose increases and when you might see better results.

"What side effects should I expect, and how long do they typically last?" Knowing that nausea, fatigue, or digestive issues are common and often temporary helps you prepare mentally.

"What side effects would be concerning enough that I should call you?" Not every side effect requires medical attention, but you need to know which ones do.

"How will we know if the medication is working for me?" Establish clear expectations about what response looks like and how long to wait before evaluating effectiveness.

"How do I store this medication? Does it need to be refrigerated?" Proper storage is essential for medication effectiveness.

"What should I do if I miss a dose?" Having a clear plan prevents anxiety if you forget an injection.

"Are there any medications or supplements I should avoid while taking this?" Some medications can interact with GLP-1s or make side effects worse.

"How often should I see you for follow-up?" Establish a monitoring schedule so you know when to expect appointments.

"What lab work will you be monitoring, and how often?" Understanding what's being checked and why helps you stay informed about your health.

"How should I adjust my eating? Are there specific nutritional guidelines I should follow?" Your doctor might have specific recommendations or might refer you to a dietitian.

Questions to Ask During Ongoing Treatment

Once you've been on the medication for a while, different questions become relevant.

"Based on my progress so far, am I responding as expected?" This helps you calibrate expectations. What feels slow to you might actually be very typical.

"Is it time to consider increasing my dose?" If your weight loss has slowed or stalled and you've been on the same dose for several weeks, a dose increase might be appropriate.

"Should we run any lab tests to check on my health?" Make sure metabolic markers like blood sugar, kidney function, and liver function are being monitored periodically.

"I've been experiencing [specific symptom]. Is this related to the medication?" Don't assume symptoms are unrelated or not worth mentioning. Let your doctor evaluate.

"My weight loss has plateaued for [X weeks/months]. What should we consider?" If progress has stalled, work with your doctor to troubleshoot whether it's medication-related, behavioral, or due to other factors.

"I'm still feeling quite hungry. Is this normal for my dose, or should we adjust?" If appetite suppression is minimal, you might need a higher dose or different medication.

"How long do you recommend I stay on this medication?" Understanding whether this is short-term treatment or long-term management helps you plan.

"What's your plan for transitioning me off this medication eventually, if that's appropriate?" Not everyone needs to stop, but if that's the plan, knowing the timeline and process helps.

Red Flags That Need Medical Attention

Most side effects from GLP-1 medications are mild and manageable. But some symptoms require immediate medical attention. Don't hesitate to contact your doctor or seek emergency care if you experience any of these.

Severe abdominal pain, especially if accompanied by nausea and vomiting, could indicate pancreatitis. This is rare but serious. The pain is usually intense and persistent in the upper abdomen and might radiate to your back.

Symptoms of gallbladder problems include severe pain in the upper right abdomen, particularly after eating fatty foods, along with nausea, vomiting, and possibly fever. Rapid weight loss increases gallstone risk.

Signs of kidney problems include decreased urination, swelling in legs or feet, unusual fatigue, or changes in urine color. GLP-1 medications can affect kidney function in rare cases, especially if you're also dehydrated.

Severe allergic reactions are rare but possible. Symptoms include difficulty breathing, swelling of face or throat, severe rash or hives, or rapid heartbeat. This requires immediate emergency care.

Signs of thyroid tumors, which are extremely rare, include a lump in your neck, persistent hoarseness, difficulty swallowing, or persistent cough. If you notice these, contact your doctor.

Severe or persistent vomiting or diarrhea that prevents you from keeping down food or fluids can lead to dehydration and requires medical attention. Don't wait days to report this.

Suicidal thoughts or severe depression should be reported immediately. Some people experience mood changes on these medications, and mental health crises require urgent intervention.

Symptoms of low blood sugar if you're also taking diabetes medications include shakiness, sweating, confusion, rapid heartbeat, or dizziness. Severe low blood sugar can be dangerous.

Vision changes, particularly in people with diabetes, should be evaluated. Rapid changes in blood sugar can temporarily affect vision, but persistent changes need assessment.

When in doubt, call your doctor's office. They can help you determine whether symptoms require immediate attention or can wait for a scheduled appointment. It's better to ask about something that turns out to be minor than to ignore something that's actually serious.

Lab Tests to Request

Regular lab work helps monitor your health while taking GLP-1 medications and during weight loss. Your doctor should be ordering these periodically, but it's reasonable to ask about them if they're not being done.

Basic metabolic panel checks kidney function, electrolytes, and blood sugar. This should be done at baseline before starting medication and periodically during treatment, perhaps every six months or annually.

Liver function tests monitor how your liver is handling the medication and weight loss. Rapid weight loss can affect liver function, so monitoring is important.

Lipid panel measures cholesterol and triglycerides. These often improve with weight loss, and tracking the improvements can be motivating. It also guides decisions about continuing or discontinuing cholesterol medications.

Hemoglobin A1C measures average blood sugar over three months. For people with diabetes or prediabetes, this should be checked regularly to see if blood sugar control is improving.

Complete blood count can identify anemia or other blood issues. This is particularly important if you're eating less and might not be getting adequate iron or other nutrients.

Thyroid function tests including TSH, free T3, and free T4 should be checked if you have symptoms suggesting thyroid problems or if weight loss is slower than expected despite good adherence.

Vitamin D levels should be checked, as many people are deficient. If you're deficient, supplementation helps with bone health, immune function, and mood.

Vitamin B12 and iron levels might be checked if you're showing symptoms of deficiency like fatigue, weakness, or cognitive issues, especially if your diet is low in meat and animal products.

For people with diabetes, checking kidney function more frequently is important since GLP-1 medications can affect kidneys and diabetes already puts kidneys at risk.

You can ask your doctor, "What lab work should we be monitoring while I'm on this medication?" or "I'd like to track my progress with lab work. What tests would be most informative?"

When Medication Adjustment Might Be Appropriate

Not everyone responds the same way to the same dose. Sometimes adjustments are needed. Here are situations where it's reasonable to discuss medication changes with your doctor.

If you've been on your current dose for at least four weeks and you're not experiencing adequate appetite suppression, a dose increase might help. You should feel noticeably less hungry than before starting the medication. If you're still frequently hungry and thinking about food constantly, the dose might be too low.

If you've lost less than 5% of your body weight after three months on what should be a therapeutic dose, and you've been adherent to dietary and exercise recommendations, the medication might not be working well for you. This is a reasonable time to discuss increasing the dose or trying a different medication.

If you started with good results but appetite has returned and weight loss has stopped or reversed, even though you're still taking the medication consistently, tolerance might be developing. Discuss whether a dose increase or medication switch makes sense.

If side effects on your current dose are intolerable and not improving over time, a dose reduction might be appropriate. Sometimes staying on a lower dose long-term is better than stopping the medication entirely because you can't tolerate the higher dose.

If you've reached your goal weight and want to maintain rather than continue losing, switching to a lower maintenance dose might be appropriate. Some people can maintain on the starting dose even though they needed higher doses for active weight loss.

If you're having repeated hypoglycemia episodes and you're also on other diabetes medications, those other medications might need adjustment. Don't adjust on your own, but definitely discuss with your doctor.

When discussing medication adjustments, come prepared with data. "I've been on this dose for six weeks. My weight has been stable for the past month. I'm tracking my food carefully and averaging 1,400 calories per day with 110 grams of protein. I'm exercising four times per week. I'm feeling quite hungry most of the time. Can we discuss whether a dose increase makes sense?"

Finding a Provider Knowledgeable About GLP-1s

Not all doctors are equally knowledgeable about GLP-1 medications for weight loss. Some are very current on the research and comfortable managing these medications. Others are less familiar and might not be the best fit for your needs.

Red flags that your provider might not be the best fit include dismissing your concerns about side effects or slow progress, being unwilling to prescribe appropriate doses, not monitoring your progress with follow-up appointments, discouraging you from taking the medication or suggesting you should just try harder with diet and exercise, not being familiar with the medications or how they work, or being defensive or dismissive when you ask questions.

If you're having these experiences, it might be time to find a different provider. You deserve a doctor who takes your weight concerns seriously, understands the medications, and works with you as a partner.

Options for finding knowledgeable providers include asking your current doctor for a referral to an endocrinologist or obesity medicine specialist, looking for medical weight loss clinics in your area that specialize in managing GLP-1 medications, searching for obesity medicine specialists through the Obesity Medicine Association directory, asking in online GLP-1 medication communities for provider recommendations in your area, or considering telehealth options if local providers aren't available or knowledgeable.

Telehealth has expanded access to GLP-1 medications significantly. Companies like Ro, Calibrate, Found, and Sequence offer medical consultations, prescriptions, and ongoing support specifically for weight loss medications. These services usually aren't covered by insurance and can be expensive, but they're an option if you can't find local providers.

When meeting with a new provider, come prepared with questions about their experience. "How many patients have you treated with GLP-1 medications for weight loss? What's your approach to titration and monitoring? How do you handle plateaus or side effects?" Their answers will tell you whether they have the expertise you need.

Insurance and Access Considerations

Cost and insurance coverage are major barriers for many people. GLP-1 medications are expensive, often $1,000 or more per month without insurance.

If you have insurance, check your specific plan's coverage. Some plans cover GLP-1s for diabetes but not for weight loss. Others cover them for weight loss only if you meet certain criteria like a BMI above a certain threshold or weight-related health conditions. Some plans don't cover them at all.

Your doctor's office can submit a prior authorization request to your insurance company. This requires documentation of your medical necessity for the medication. Having documented weight-related health conditions like high blood pressure, diabetes, or sleep apnea can strengthen the case.

If insurance denies coverage, you can appeal. Your doctor can write a letter explaining why the medication is medically necessary. Sometimes appeals are successful, though the process can be time-consuming.

Manufacturer savings programs can significantly reduce cost. Novo Nordisk offers savings cards for Ozempic and Wegovy. Eli Lilly has programs for Mounjaro and Zepbound. These programs can reduce your out-of-pocket cost to as little as $25 per month, though eligibility requirements vary and they typically don't work with government insurance like Medicare or Medicaid.

Compounding pharmacies make their own versions

of semaglutide and tirzepatide, usually at lower cost than brand-name medications. This has become more common during shortages. Compounded versions cost $200 to $400 per month typically. However, compounded medications aren't FDA-approved, quality can vary between pharmacies, and there are safety considerations. Discuss with your doctor whether compounded versions are appropriate for you.

If cost is prohibitive, discuss alternatives with your doctor. Other weight loss medications might be more affordable. Or you might be able to use lifestyle modifications alone, though outcomes typically aren't as good without medication.

Ask your doctor's office about patient assistance programs. Pharmaceutical companies sometimes have programs for people who can't afford medications. Eligibility is usually based on income and lack of insurance.

Questions to ask about cost and access include "Does my insurance cover this medication? If not, what are my options?" "Are there manufacturer savings programs I can use?" "If I can't afford the brand-name medication, are compounded versions a safe alternative?" "How much will this cost me per month after insurance and savings programs?" "If I have to stop the medication due to cost, what's the plan for maintaining my weight loss?"

Preparing for Appointments
To make the most of your time with your healthcare

provider, come prepared.

Bring your tracking data for at least the past week, preferably longer. Food logs, weight records, exercise logs, any symptoms you've been experiencing.

Write down specific questions in order of importance. Start with the most critical questions in case you run out of time.

Know your medication details. What dose you're taking, how long you've been on that dose, when you last increased.

If you've made any changes to diet, exercise, or other medications since your last appointment, be ready to discuss those.

Think about your goals for the appointment. Are you there for routine monitoring? To discuss a specific concern? To request a dose adjustment? Knowing what you want to accomplish helps focus the conversation.

If you're seeing a new provider, bring a list of all your medications, supplements, and medical conditions. Bring relevant medical records if they're not already in the system.

Your Role in Your Own Care

Remember that you're an active participant in your healthcare, not a passive recipient. Your doctor has medical expertise, but you're the expert on your own body and experience.

Speak up when something doesn't feel right. Advocate for yourself when you need more support or different approaches.

Be honest about challenges you're facing. Ask questions until you understand.

At the same time, trust your healthcare provider's expertise. They've gone through years of training and have experience treating many patients. When they make recommendations based on medical knowledge, take them seriously even if they're not what you wanted to hear.

The best patient-provider relationship is a partnership. You bring information about your experience, adherence, and concerns. Your provider brings medical knowledge, monitoring, and treatment decisions. Together, you work toward your health goals.

Conclusion
Your Path Forward

You've made it through sixteen chapters of information, strategies, and troubleshooting advice. That's a lot to absorb. If you're feeling a bit overwhelmed, that's completely normal. You don't need to implement everything at once. In fact, trying to do everything perfectly from day one is a recipe for burnout.

Let me bring this all back to something simple and actionable.

What Matters Most

If you take away nothing else from this book, remember these core principles.

GLP-1 medications are powerful tools, but they're not magic. They suppress appetite remarkably well for most people, but appetite suppression alone doesn't guarantee weight loss. You still need to actually be in a calorie deficit. You still need adequate protein to protect muscle. You still need to move your body. The medication makes all of these things dramatically easier, but it doesn't eliminate the need for them.

Protein is non-negotiable. If you only focus on one nutritional factor, make it protein. Aim for at least 100 grams per day, more if you're larger or very active. Eat protein first at every meal. Use protein shakes if needed. This single habit will protect your muscle, support your metabolism, and improve your results more than almost anything else.

Resistance training matters more than you think. Lift weights, use resistance bands, or do challenging bodyweight exercises at least twice per week. This preserves muscle during weight loss and completely changes your body composition. The difference between losing weight with and without resistance training is dramatic.

Your body is complex. Genetics, thyroid function, hormones, stress, sleep, medications you're taking, and dozens of other factors affect how you respond to GLP-1 medications. If progress is slower than expected, don't immediately blame yourself. Work systematically through potential issues with your doctor.

Slower is often better. Rapid weight loss feels exciting, but it often comes with excessive muscle loss, more severe metabolic adaptation, and higher likelihood of regain. Losing one to two pounds per week is actually ideal for most people. Be patient with the process.

What Success Really Looks Like

Success isn't just a number on the scale. It's not fitting into a specific size of jeans or looking a certain way in photos. Real success is multifaceted.

Success is improving your health markers. Lower blood pressure, better blood sugar control, improved cholesterol, reduced inflammation. These changes extend your life and improve your quality of life regardless of what the scale says.

Success is feeling better in your body. Having more energy to play with your kids or grandkids. Walking without getting winded. Sleeping better. Moving more easily. These day-to-day improvements in how you feel and function matter enormously.

Success is building sustainable habits. Learning to prioritize protein. Exercising consistently. Managing stress. Getting adequate sleep. Creating a lifestyle that supports your health long-term. These habits serve you whether you're actively losing weight or maintaining.

Success is developing a healthier relationship with food. Moving away from all-or-nothing thinking. Letting go of guilt and shame around eating. Finding balance between enjoying food and nourishing your body. This psychological shift often matters more than any specific dietary strategy.

Success is maintaining whatever weight loss you achieve. Keeping off even 5 to 10% of your body weight produces meaningful health benefits. You don't have to reach some ideal weight to be successful. Maintaining a lower weight than where you started is a victory.

When Things Don't Go as Planned

Not everything will go smoothly. You'll have weeks where the scale doesn't move. You'll have periods where motivation is low. You'll slip back into old habits sometimes. You might experience frustrating side effects. You might not lose as much weight as you hoped or as quickly as you expected.

All of that is normal. It doesn't mean you're failing. It doesn't mean the medication isn't working. It doesn't mean you should give up.

When progress stalls or challenges arise, go back to the basics. Are you tracking food accurately? Are you hitting your protein target? Are you exercising consistently? Are you sleeping enough? Are you managing stress? Usually, tightening up one or two of these foundational habits gets things moving again.

If the basics are solid and you're still struggling, work through the troubleshooting strategies in this book. Check for metabolic issues. Evaluate medications that might be interfering. Consider whether lifestyle factors like stress or alcohol are holding you back. Look at whether emotional eating or old patterns have crept back in.

And if you've tried everything and you're still not getting results, get professional help. See an endocrinologist, work with a registered dietitian, talk to a therapist who specializes in eating behaviors. There's no prize for figuring everything out alone. Using available resources and expertise is smart, not weak.

The Long View

This isn't a sprint. It's not even really a marathon. It's a fundamental shift in how you live your life. That shift takes time, practice, and patience.

You didn't gain weight overnight, and you won't lose it overnight. You didn't develop unhealthy habits in a few weeks, and you won't build new healthy habits in a few weeks. Give yourself time to learn, adjust, and grow.

Some people stay on GLP-1 medications indefinitely. Others transition off after reaching their goals. Either approach is fine. There's no right answer. Do what works for you, what you can sustain, and what supports your health long-term.

Whether you stay on medication or not, the habits you build now will serve you for the rest of your life. The protein-focused eating. The regular exercise. The attention to sleep and stress management. The self-awareness around emotional eating. These are skills that improve your health and quality of life regardless of medication status.

You Can Do This

If you're reading this book, you've already taken an

important step. You're being proactive about your health. You're seeking information. You're willing to do the work. Those qualities predict success more than any medication or strategy.

Will it always be easy? No. Will you have setbacks? Probably. Will you sometimes feel frustrated or discouraged? Almost certainly. But will you get results if you stay consistent and patient? Yes.

Thousands of people have used GLP-1 medications to lose significant weight and improve their health. You can be one of them. The medication gives you a powerful advantage. The strategies in this book give you a roadmap. Your consistency and commitment will get you there.

You're not alone in this journey. Millions of people are taking these medications. Countless others have struggled with weight and found solutions. Your healthcare providers are there to support you. Online and in-person communities can provide encouragement and practical advice. And this book will be here whenever you need to reference specific strategies or troubleshoot specific issues.

Final Thoughts

Be kind to yourself. You're doing something difficult. Change is hard. Weight loss is complicated. Bodies are complex. You won't do everything perfectly, and that's okay. Progress, not perfection, is the goal.

Celebrate your victories, big and small. Lost five pounds? That's real progress. Went to the gym three times this week? That's an accomplishment. Hit your protein target every day? You should feel proud. These wins add up to significant change over time.

Stay curious and flexible. If something isn't working, be willing to try a different approach. If you discover new strategies that work for you, incorporate them. This journey is yours to customize based on what your body responds to and what fits your life.

Keep your why visible. Remember why you started this journey. Write it down. Look at it when things get hard. Whether your motivation is health, longevity, energy, confidence, or being able to do activities you love, keep that reason front and center.

And finally, know that whatever happens with your weight, you are valuable. Your worth isn't determined by a number on a scale or the size of your clothes. You're working on your health because you deserve to feel good and live well, not because you need to earn your value by changing your body.

You've got this. The information is here. The tools are available. The path forward is clear. Now it's time to take that next step.

Good luck on your journey.

About the Author

David Brant is a personal trainer based in Vancouver, British Columbia, Canada. With over two decades of experience in fitness and wellness, he has helped countless clients achieve their health goals through personalized training and evidence-based guidance. David's practical approach to nutrition and fitness is informed by years of real-world experience working with people navigating their unique wellness journeys.